Improve Your Flexibility
& Fitness with the...

Ultimate Guide to
STRETCHING
& FLEXIBILITY

...for all ages, all sports
and all fitness levels.

Brad Walker

What are the experts saying about the Ultimate Guide to Stretching & Flexibility? *(Formally the Stretching Handbook)*

"An excellent, important guide to optimum health and peak performance. Read, learn, implement and enjoy the benefits of wellness and enhanced quality of life."

Dr Denis Waitley (PhD)
Author & Past Chairman - US Olympic Committee

"Up to now, while there has been a plethora of books about, 'How to...' 'The benefits of...' exercise, there has not been much advice offered regarding stretching. I believe your book fills that gap very well. Stretching is a very important and often neglected part of exercise. I congratulate you on your efforts and look forward to recommending your publication to my patients."

Dr John Flynn
Sports Medicine Australia

"The acceptance of the importance of flexibility and stretching for sport is commonplace, but appropriate and accessible information for athletes and coaches to use is not always easy to find. The Stretching Handbook is designed to be a very portable and quick reference for athletes and coaches rather than an academic reference. To this end it is a very practical text with concise chapters written in an easy-to-read manner but without being punctuated by research findings or scientific references. Overall, it is well laid out, user-friendly and very suitable for athletes and developing coaches. It is a welcome addition to the limited number of texts that deal with stretching for sport."

Angela Calder
Performance Consultant - Australian Institute of Sport

"The Stretching Handbook has given me a greater understanding and appreciation of the importance of stretching. After reading The Stretching Handbook my coach and I decided to write specific stretching time into my program, thus taking stretching far more seriously. Thanks for allowing me to read The Stretching Handbook. It is definitely a book that anybody wanting to exercise and even more so, elite athletes, should have by their side."

Greg Bennett
World Champion Triathlete

"The Stretching Handbook provides a comprehensive guide to the art of stretching. The detailed photographic catalogue of stretching exercises serves as an easy-to-follow reference guide for athletes and coaches alike."

Wayne Pearce
Coach - Balmain Tigers RLFC

"Stretching is an important part of any exercise program to help prevent injury and to increase flexibility. The Stretching Handbook is a clear, concise guide to stretches for all areas of the body."
Bob Fulton
Coach - Manly Sea Eagles RLFC & Australian Team Coach

"The Stretching Handbook is a useful resource for all coaches. The photographs and explanations are clear and concise. A much needed resource."

Janet Bothwell
National Director of Coaching - Netball Australian

"A thoroughly professional and comprehensive book on a subject that previously was very much neglected. It will play an important role for coaches and athletes in preparation for their specific sports. The Stretching Handbook is a must for anybody in the health and fitness industry."

Tony Green
Strength & Conditioning Coach - Gold Coast Chargers RLFC

"Overall The Stretching Handbook is a great resource for coaches and athletes. It offers a quick and easy reference to stretches for all areas of the body. Its size is an added bonus, making it easy to fit into a bag or back pocket."

Jill McIntosh
Coach - Australian Netball Team

"A comprehensive, helpful and easy-to-read publication. Great for amateurs and professionals."

Frank Farina
Australian Socceroo
Player / Coach - Brisbane Strikers

"As a sportsman and now in my role offering improved health and preventative health care, I see this as a very practical tool for people of all walks of life. May it encourage all people to stretch to new heights of health and well being."

Brendan Long (B.Ed.)
General Manager - Camp Eden Health Retreat

Dedicated to JC: It's all you!

Walker, Bradley E., 1971
Ultimate Guide to Stretching & Flexibility *(Formally the Stretching Handbook)*, 3rd Edition

ISBN: 978-0-9581093-5-2 (Spiral bound)

Copyright © 2011, 2007, 1998, 1997 The Stretching Institute™
All rights reserved. Except under conditions described in the copyright act, no part of this publication may in any form or by any means (electronic, mechanical, micro copying, photocopying, recording or otherwise) be reproduced, stored in a retrieval system or transmitted without prior written permission from the copyright owner. Inquires should be addressed to the publisher.

Warning
The stretching exercises presented in this publication are intended as an educational resource and are not intended as a substitute for proper medical advice. Please consult your physician, physical therapist or sports coach before performing any of the stretching exercises described in this publication, particularly if you are pregnant, elderly or have any chronic or recurring muscle or joint pain. Discontinue any exercise that causes you pain or severe discomfort and consult a medical expert.

The Stretching Institute™
Website: TheStretchingInstitute.com
Address: 4747 36th Street, Suite 3208
                Long Island City, NY 11101
                UNITED STATES
Telephone: +1 877-580-7771

Contents

Introduction	**7**

Chapter 1 – An Overview of Stretching and Flexibility   **9**
What is flexibility?
What is stretching?
Fitness and flexibility
The dangers of poor flexibility
How is flexibility restricted?
Flexibility and the aging process

Chapter 2 – The Benefits of Stretching   **13**
Improved range of motion (ROM)
Increased power
Reduced delayed onset muscle soreness
Reduced fatigue
Added benefits
Why is there so much confusion about stretching?
Stretching is not a quick fix

Chapter 3 – A Stretching Story   **17**

Chapter 4 – The Types of Stretching   **19**
Static Stretches
    Static Stretching
    Passive (or Assisted) Stretching
    Active Stretching
    PNF Stretching
    Isometric Stretching
Dynamic Stretches
    Ballistic Stretching
    Dynamic Stretching
    Active Isolated Stretching
    Resistance Stretching and Loaded Stretching

Chapter 5 – The Rules for Safe Stretching   **25**
There is no such thing as a good or bad stretch!
The specific requirements of the individual

Warm-up prior to stretching
Stretch before and after exercise
Stretch all major muscles and their opposing muscle groups
Stretch gently and slowly
Stretch ONLY to the point of tension
Breathe slowly and easily while stretching
An example

Chapter 6 – How to Stretch Properly   31
When to stretch?
What type of stretching?
Hold, Count, Repeat
Sequence
Posture
How to use stretching as part of the warm-up
What has science got to say?
The greatest misconception
What conclusions can we make?

Chapter 7 – Flexibility Testing   37
Sit and Reach Test
Shoulder Flexibility Test
Hamstring Flexibility Test

Chapter 8 – 135 Unique Stretching Exercises   41
Neck and Shoulders   45
Arms and Chest   55
Stomach   65
Back and Sides   69
Hips and Buttocks   83
Quadriceps   91
Hamstrings   97
Adductors   107
Abductors   113
Upper Calves   119
Lower Calves and Achilles   125
Shins, Ankles, Feet and Toes   131

Top 5 Stretches for each Sport   135
Top 5 Stretches for each Sports Injury   137
Resources   139

Introduction

In the late 1980's and early 1990's I was competing as a professional triathlete and working in the sports coaching industry. I had the pleasure of working with a number of high profile coaches, athletes and sports doctors, and I started to notice a common theme among the injured athletes that I saw: A lack of flexibility.

At university I dedicated a large portion of my time to the study of stretching and flexibility training, and wherever possible chose the topic for my assignments and research papers.

Then in 1992 I was fortunate enough to work with an exceptional sports coach by the name of Col Stewart. Col is one of those rare coaches who can take just about any sport, and devise a specific training program that always produces outstanding improvements for the athlete. His coaching is largely responsible for the success of many of his world champion athletes: Including his son, Miles Stewart (World Triathlon Champion); Mick Doohan (World 500cc Motorcycle Champion); and countless others from sports as diverse as roller-skating, squash, and cycling.

During my time under his tuition, I noticed that his athletes were able to remain injury free while sustaining training loads that would cripple the average athlete. And one of the keys to his athletes' success was stretching.

I was convinced that improved flexibility through the proper use of stretching was a key component to improving athletic performance and reducing susceptibility to sports injury. The problem was; I could not find a publication that was as serious about stretching as I was.

By 1995 I had become frustrated with the lack of information about stretching and was desperately seeking a comprehensive guide to flexibility training: A book that took stretching and flexibility seriously, with a detailed list and picture of every possible sports-related stretch a person could do. In my search I found many books where stretching got a mention, but nothing more than a page or two of vague generalizations and a few stick figures performing some very basic stretches. So I decided to stop searching and start writing.

In 1997, when the first edition of the Ultimate Guide to Stretching & Flexibility *(Formally the Stretching Handbook)* was released, there was only one other publication entirely dedicated to the topic of stretching. Today there are dozens, but the Ultimate Guide to Stretching & Flexibility continues to stand alone as the most user-friendly resource on stretching and flexibility training for athletes, coaches, trainers, therapists and health care professionals.

The Ultimate Guide to Stretching & Flexibility is written as an easy-to-use, quick reference guide so you don't have to read it from cover to cover to take advantage of the information within. It contains 135 unique stretching exercises for every muscle group in the body and has been designed so you can carry it with you and refer to it often. This is a back-pocket handbook not a sit-on-the-shelf text book.

If you want information on stretches for the back, look under that section; if you want to know what stretching can do for you, have a read through some of the benefits in chapter 2; or if you want to make sure you are stretching properly, refer to the *Rules for Safe Stretching* in chapter 5.

Whether you are a professional athlete or a fitness enthusiast; a sports coach or personal trainer; a physical therapist or sports doctor, the Ultimate Guide to Stretching & Flexibility will benefit you.

Yours in sport

Brad Walker

AKA the Stretch Coach
And Founder of...
The Stretching Institute

Chapter 1
An Overview of Stretching and Flexibility

What is flexibility?
Flexibility is commonly described as the range of motion, or movement, (ROM) around a particular joint or set of joints. In layman's terms; how far we can reach, bend and turn.

When improving flexibility is the goal, the muscles and their fascia (sheath) should be the major focus of flexibility training. While bones, joints, ligaments, tendons and skin do contribute to overall flexibility, we have limited control over these factors.

What is stretching?
Stretching, as it relates to physical health and fitness, is the process of placing particular parts of the body into a position that will lengthen the muscles and their associated soft tissues.

Upon undertaking a regular stretching program a number of changes begin to occur within the body and specifically within the muscles themselves. Other tissues that begin to adapt to the stretching process include the fascia, tendons, skin and scar tissue.

Fitness and flexibility
An individuals' physical fitness depends upon a number of components, and flexibility is only one of these. Although flexibility is a vital part of physical fitness it is important to see it as only *one spoke in the fitness wheel*. Other components include strength, power, speed, endurance, balance, agility, skill and co-ordination.

Although different sports require different levels of each fitness component it is essential to plan a regular exercise or training program that covers all the components of physical fitness.

Rugby and Gridiron for example, rely heavily on strength and power; however the exclusion of skill drills and flexibility training could lead to injury and poor performance. Strength and flexibility are of prime importance to a gymnast, but a balanced training program would also improve power, speed and endurance.

The same is true for each individual, while some people may be naturally strong or flexible it would be foolish for such a person to completely ignore the other components of physical fitness. And just because an individual exhibits good flexibility at one joint or muscle group does not mean that the entire individual will be flexible. Therefore, flexibility can be assessed according to a specific muscle group, a specific joint or the specific requirements of a particular sport.

The dangers of poor flexibility

Tight, stiff muscles limit normal range of motion. In some cases, a lack of flexibility can be a major contributing factor to muscle and joint pain. In the extreme, a lack of flexibility can mean it is difficult, for example, to bend down or look over the shoulder.

Tight, stiff muscles interfere with proper muscle action. If the muscles cannot contract and relax efficiently, decreased performance and a lack of muscle movement control will result. Short, tight muscles can also cause a loss of strength and power during physical activity.

In a very small percentage of cases tight, stiff muscles can even restrict blood circulation. Good blood circulation is vitally important to ensure the muscles receive adequate amounts of oxygen and nutrients. Poor circulation can result in increased muscle fatigue and ultimately, the ability to recover from strenuous exercise and the muscles repair process is impeded.

Any one of these factors can greatly increase the chance of becoming injured. Together they present a package that includes muscular discomfort; loss of performance; an increased risk of soft tissue injury; and a greater likelihood of repeated injury.

How is flexibility restricted?

The muscular system needs to be flexible to achieve peak performance and stretching is the most effective way of developing and retaining flexible muscles and joints. However, a number of other factors also contribute to a decrease in flexibility.

Flexibility, or range of motion, can be restricted by both internal and external factors. Internal factors such as bones, ligaments, muscle bulk, muscle length, tendons and skin all restrict the amount of movement at any particular joint. As an example, the human leg cannot extend forward beyond a straight position because of the structure of the bones and ligaments that make up the knee joint.

External factors such as age, gender, temperature, restrictive clothing and of course any injury or disability will also have an effect on ones flexibility.

Flexibility and the aging process

It is no secret that with each passing year muscles and joints become more stiff and tight. This is part of the ageing process and is caused by a combination of physical degeneration and inactivity. Although we cannot halt the aging process completely, this should not mean giving up on trying to improve flexibility and fitness.

Age should not be an excuse that prevents one from living a fit and active lifestyle, but certain precautions should be taken as we get older. (Refer to the *Rules for Safe Stretching* in chapter 5 for more information.)

Chapter 2
The Benefits of Stretching

Stretching is a simple and effective activity that helps to enhance athletic performance, decrease the likelihood of sports injury and minimize muscle soreness. But how specifically is this accomplished?

Improved range of motion (ROM)
By placing particular parts of the body in certain positions, we are able to increase the length of the muscles and their associated soft tissues. As a result of this, a reduction in general muscle tension is achieved and range of motion is increased.

By increasing range of motion we are increasing the distance our limbs can move before damage occurs to the muscles and other soft tissues. For example, the muscles and tendons in the back of the legs are put under great strain when kicking a ball. Therefore, the more flexible and pliable those muscles are, the greater the range of motion and the further the leg can travel forward before a strain or injury occurs to them.

The benefits of an extended range of motion include: increased comfort; a greater ability to move freely; and a lessening of the susceptibility to soft tissue injuries like muscle and tendon strains.

Increased power
There is a dangerous stretching myth that says, *if you stretch too much you will lose both joint stability and muscle power*. This is untrue, (as long as *The Rules for Safe Stretching* in chapter 5 are observed). By increasing muscle length and range of motion we are increasing the distance over which the muscles are able to contract. This results in a potential increase to the muscles power and therefore increases athletic ability, while also leading to an improvement in dynamic balance, or the ability to control the muscles.

Reduced delayed onset muscle soreness
Most have experienced what happens when we go for a run or to the gym for the first time after an extended break. The following day the muscles are tight, sore, stiff, and it is usually hard to even walk down a flight of stairs. This soreness that usually accompanies strenuous physical activity is referred to as delayed onset muscle soreness (DOMS). This soreness is the

result of micro tears, (minute tears within the muscle fibers), blood pooling and accumulated waste products, such as lactic acid. Stretching, as part of an effective cool-down, helps to alleviate this soreness by lengthening the individual muscle fibers; increasing blood circulation; and removing waste products.

Reduced fatigue

Fatigue is a major problem for everyone, especially those who exercise. It results in a decrease in both physical and mental performance. Increased flexibility through stretching can help prevent the effects of fatigue by taking pressure off the working muscles, (the agonist).

For every muscle in the body there is an opposite or opposing muscle, (the antagonist). If the opposing muscles are more flexible, the working muscles do not have to exert as much force against the opposing muscles. Therefore each movement of the working muscles actually takes less effort.

Added benefits

Along with the benefits listed above, a regular stretching program will also help to improve posture; develop body awareness; improve co-ordination; promote circulation; increase energy; and improve relaxation and stress relief.

Why is there so much confusion about stretching?

If improving flexibility will result in all the benefits listed above, why is it common to hear reports that say; *stretching should be avoided?*

The study of stretching and flexibility training really has a long way to go. If someone told the average sports coach or personal trainer that bicep curls are the best exercise; the reply would be "please explain!" *The best for what? The best for whom? What type of bicep curl? And when are they the best?* The person making this sort of claim would be dismissed as ignorant and un-learned.

But these are the same sort of statements that I hear about stretching every day. And the problem is; that same sports coach or personal trainer who questioned the statement about bicep curls; accepts by blind faith that these statements about stretching are true, without giving them a second thought.

Statements like: *The best type of stretching is dynamic stretching. Never do this stretch. This is the best stretch. Don't stretch before exercise.*

The Benefits of Stretching

These ridiculous statements are causing a lot of confusion about the topic of stretching and causing some people to abandon stretching altogether.

These unqualified statements, like the ones above, should not be made without fully disclosing all the parameters involved. For example, I recently heard a lecturer make the comment... "*The best time to stretch is 2 hours after exercise.*" This statement needs to be questioned.

Stretch for what: To improve flexibility; to improve recovery; to avoid injury? And for whom: For athletes; for sedentary people; for those looking to improve flexibility; for those looking to improve performance; for someone recovering from an injury? And what type of stretching is he talking about: Static stretching; PNF stretching; dynamic stretching; AI stretching?

A new level of professionalism is required for the topic of stretching and flexibility training. The professionalism and competency of the strength training industry has developed monumentally over the last 20 years and it is time that the flexibility industry does the same. More questions need to be asked and current theories need to be expanded and explained in more detail.

The bottom line is: Stretching is beneficial, when used correctly. Remember, stretching is just one very important component that assists to reduce the risk of injury and improve athletic performance. The best results are achieved when stretching is used in combination with other injury reduction techniques and conditioning exercises.

Stretching is not a quick fix

Even with all the benefits listed earlier, stretching is not a quick fix. No one is going to do a few stretches before they exercise and magically become a better athlete or totally resilient to injury.

Just the same as doing three sets of lunges before playing basketball will not make someone a better basketball player, or doing three sets of bicep curls before playing tennis will not make them a better tennis player, the same applies to stretching. Doing three sets of hamstring stretches before running onto the sports field will do very little, if anything for anyone.

This is where a number of recent studies have fallen short. In an attempt to measure the benefits of stretching, researchers have tried to use stretching in the same way as the examples above. They have tried to measure the effects of doing a few stretches before playing sport, and when the results of their research suggest that no benefit was gained, they make the wrong assumption that stretching is a waste of time.

Stretching was never meant to be used in this way, and if anyone makes the claim that doing a few stretches before you exercise will make you a better athlete or less susceptible to injury, they are incorrect.

The benefits of stretching are only attained when flexibility training is applied professionally and diligently over an extended period of time; just the same as a weight loss program, or strength training program. No one expects to lose weight after eating one healthy meal, or grow big muscles after doing one workout in the gym.

Stretching is beneficial, when used correctly.

Chapter 3
A Stretching Story

Once upon a time there was an eager, young athlete ready to take on the world. He trained hard, ate right, got lots of rest and did all the things a budding young athlete should do.

His specialty was the 10 km run and he was quite good too. His personal best was 32 minutes and 4 seconds, which is pretty good for a seventeen year old kid. But he longed to break the 30 minute barrier; he had tried everything but nothing seemed to work.

His training program was well structured and very professional. He was disciplined and rarely wavered from his set training schedule. He incorporated long runs, tempo runs, interval training, weight training in the gym, hill running, cross country running, deep water running and various other training methods to try and improve his personal best. He even bought a mountain bike to introduce cross training into his program.

He always ate right, took extra vitamins and minerals to supplement his diet and always made sure that he drank plenty of water. He made sure he was well rested and even got the occasional massage to help his legs recover.

I met our budding young athlete at a local fun-run where he had a good race and achieved a time that most people would be happy with. Although it was close to his personal best, it was still nowhere near his goal of breaking 30 minutes.

We got to talking and I could tell he was disheartened and frustrated. He explained to me that he had tried everything and nothing he did seemed to improve his personal best. I asked if he would mind if I attended one of his training sessions and he welcomed the idea of getting some fresh advice.

As it turned out, the next session that I could get to was an interval session at the local 400 meter track. As I arrived he was just finishing his warm-up with a few run-throughs. For this session he was doing eight, 400 meter intervals with plenty of rest in between each one.

As soon as he started the first interval I could tell what was wrong. His hamstring and hip muscles were so tight that they restricted the normal range of motion of his legs to the extent that they shortened his stride length. For a tall guy with long legs his stride length was atrociously short.

After he finished his cool-down I asked him if he ever did any stretching. He replied quite honestly by saying he did none at all. Just to be sure we did a few flexibility tests for his back, hamstrings and calves. From these it was quite obvious that his flexibility was a major limiting factor in achieving his goal.

I went on to explain how his lack of flexibility was contributing to a shortened stride length, which in turn was making it difficult to improve his personal best time. Armed with this new bit of hope he eagerly wanted advice on how to incorporate stretching into his training program.

We sat down together and reviewed his training program for the next two weeks. We decided not to make any changes to the program itself, but simply add a general stretching workout to each session. The only advice I gave him was to add a few minutes of dynamic stretching before each training session, add another 15 minutes of static stretching after each session and at least 30 minutes of static stretching before going to bed each night.

The results did not happen straight away, but within two weeks his general flexibility improved considerably. We then incorporated a number of specific stretches to further increase the flexibility of his back, hamstrings, hips and calves.

The improvements over the next couple of months were remarkable. Not only did his times improve but his running style and technique also improved considerably.

The last time I spoke with our budding young athlete he still had not achieved his 30 minute goal, but his 400 meter time had dropped to less than 60 seconds. His 5 km personal best was right on 15 minutes and his 10 km personal best was now just under 31 minutes. I am positive it is only a matter of time before he achieves his goal of breaking 30 minutes for 10 km.

Remember, that except for adding stretching to his program, nothing else changed. We did not add anything to his program and we did not take anything away. All we did was incorporate a few basic stretching exercises as a regular part of his training and the results were remarkable.

Do not make the mistake of thinking that something as simple as stretching will not be effective. Stretching is a vital part of any exercise program and should be looked upon as being as important as any other part of your health and fitness.

Chapter 4
The Types of Stretching

Stretching is slightly more technical than swinging a leg over a park bench. There are methods and techniques that will maximize the benefits and minimize the risk of injury. In this chapter we will look at the different types of stretching, the particular benefits, risks and uses, plus a description of how each type is performed.

Just as there are many different ways to strength train, there are also many different ways to stretch. However, it is important to note that although there are many different ways to stretch, no one way, or no one type of stretching is better than another. Each type has its own advantages and disadvantages, and the key to getting the most out of stretching lies in being able to match the right type of stretching to the purpose, or goal trying to be achieved.

For example; PNF and passive stretching are great for creating permanent improvements in flexibility, but they are not very useful for warming up or preparing the body for activity. Dynamic stretching, on the other hand, is great for warming up but can be dangerous if used in the initial stages of injury rehabilitation.

Although there are many different ways to stretch, they can all be grouped into one of two categories; static or dynamic.

Static Stretches

The term static stretches refers to stretching exercises that are performed without movement. In other words, the individual gets into the stretch position and holds the stretch for a specific amount of time. Listed below are five different types of static stretching exercises.

Static Stretching
Static stretching is performed by placing the body into a position whereby the muscle (or group of muscles) to be stretched is under tension. Both the antagonist, or opposing muscle group and the agonist, or muscles to be stretched are relaxed. Then slowly and cautiously the body is moved to increase the tension on the stretched muscle (or group of muscles). At this point the position is held or maintained to allow the muscles to relax and lengthen.

The stretch to the right is a classic example of a static stretch in which the opposing muscles and the hamstring and back muscles are relaxed.

A minimum hold time of about 20 seconds is required for the muscles to relax and start to lengthen, while diminishing returns are experienced after 45 to 60 seconds.

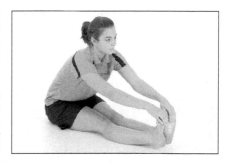

Static stretching is a very safe and effective form of stretching with a limited threat of injury. It is a good choice for beginners and sedentary individuals.

Passive (or Assisted) Stretching

This form of stretching is very similar to static stretching; however another person or apparatus is used to help further stretch the muscles. Due to the greater force applied to the muscles, this form of stretching can be slightly more hazardous. Therefore it is very important that any apparatus used is both solid and stable. When using a partner it is imperative that no jerky or bouncing force is applied to the stretched muscles. So, choose a partner carefully; the partner is responsible for the safety of the muscles and joints while you are performing the stretching exercises.

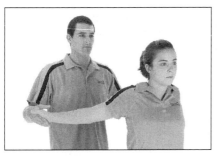

The stretch on the left is an example of a passive stretch in which a partner is used to stretch the chest and shoulder muscles.

Passive stretching is useful in helping to attain a greater range of motion, but carries with it a slightly higher risk of injury. It can also be used effectively as part of a rehabilitation program or as part of a cool-down.

Active Stretching

Active stretching is performed without any aid or assistance from an external force. This form of stretching involves using only the strength of the opposing muscles (antagonist) to generate a stretch within the target muscle group (agonist). The contraction of the opposing muscles helps to relax the stretched muscles.

A classic example of an active stretch is one where an individual raises one leg straight out in front, as high as possible, and then maintains that fixed position without any assistance from a partner or object.

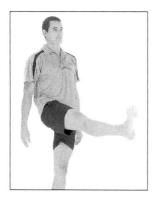

Active stretching is useful as a rehabilitation tool and very effective as a form of conditioning before moving onto dynamic stretches. This type of stretching exercise is usually quite difficult to hold and maintain for long periods of time and therefore the stretch position is usually only held for 10 to 15 seconds.

PNF Stretching

PNF stretching (*Proprioceptive Neuromuscular Facilitation*), sometimes referred to as *Facilitated Stretching*, is a more advanced form of flexibility training that involves both the stretching and contracting of the muscle group being targeted. PNF stretching was originally developed as a form of rehabilitation and for that function it is very effective. It is also excellent for targeting specific muscle groups, and as well as increasing flexibility, it also improves muscular strength.

There are many different variations of the PNF stretching principle and sometimes it is referred to as Contract-Relax stretching or Hold-Relax stretching. Post Isometric Relaxation (PIR) is another variation of the PNF technique.

To perform a PNF stretch, the area to be stretched is positioned so that the muscle (or group of muscles) is under tension. The individual then contracts the stretched muscle group for 5 to 6 seconds while a partner (or immovable object) applies sufficient resistance to inhibit movement. The force of contraction should be relative to the level of conditioning. The

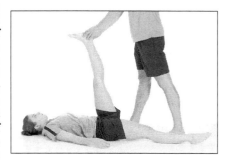

contracted muscle group is then relaxed and a controlled stretch is immediately applied for about 30 seconds. The athlete is then allowed 30 seconds to recover and the process is repeated 2 to 4 times.

Information differs slightly about timing recommendations for PNF stretching. Although there are conflicting responses to the questions; *for how long should I contract the muscle group* and *for how long should I rest between each stretch*, it is my professional opinion, that through a study of research literature and personal experience, the previous timing recommendations provide the maximum benefits from PNF stretching.

Isometric Stretching

Isometric stretching is a form of passive stretching similar to PNF stretching, but the contractions are held for a longer period of time. Isometric stretching places high demands on the stretched muscles and is not recommended for children or adolescents who are still growing. Other recommendations include allowing at least 48 hours rest between isometric stretching sessions and performing only one isometric stretching exercise per muscle group in a session.

A classic example of how isometric stretching is used is the *Leaning Heel-back Calf Stretch* to the right. In this stretch the participant stands upright, leans forward towards a wall and then places one foot as far from the wall as is comfortable while making sure that the heel remains on the ground. In this position, the participant contracts the calf muscles as if trying to raise the heel off the ground.

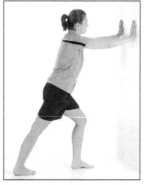

To perform an isometric stretch; assume the position of the passive stretch and then contract the stretched muscle for 10 to 15 seconds. Be sure that all movement of the limb is prevented. Then relax the muscle for at least 20 seconds. This procedure should be repeated 2 to 5 times.

Dynamic Stretches

The term dynamic stretches refers to stretching exercises that are performed with movement. In other words, the individual uses a swinging or bouncing movement to extend their range of motion and flexibility. Listed below are four different types of dynamic stretching exercises.

Ballistic Stretching
Ballistic stretching is an outdated form of stretching that uses momentum generated by rapid swinging, bouncing and rebounding movements to force a body part past its normal range of motion.

The risks associated with ballistic stretching far outweigh the gains, especially when greater gains can be achieved by using other forms of stretching like dynamic stretching and PNF stretching. Other than potential injury, the main disadvantage of ballistic stretching is that it fails to allow the stretched muscle time to adapt to the stretched position and instead may cause the muscle to tighten up by repeatedly triggering the stretch reflex, (*discussed in chapter 5*).

Dynamic Stretching
Unlike ballistic stretching, dynamic stretching uses a controlled, soft bounce or swinging movement to move a particular body part to the limit of its range of motion. The force of the bounce or swing is gradually increased but should never become radical or uncontrolled.

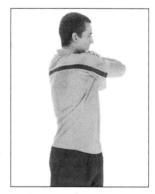

Do not confuse dynamic stretching with ballistic stretching. Dynamic stretching is slow, gentle and very purposeful. At no time during dynamic stretching should a body part be forced past the joints normal range of motion. Ballistic stretching, on the other hand, is much more aggressive and its very purpose is to force the body part beyond the limit of its normal range of motion.

Active Isolated Stretching
Active isolated (AI) stretching is a form of stretching developed by Aaron L. Mattes, and is sometimes referred to as *The Mattes Method*. It works by contracting the antagonist, or opposing muscle group, which forces the

stretched muscle group to relax. The procedure for performing an AI stretch is as follows.

1. Choose the muscle group to be stretched and then get into a position to begin the stretch.
2. Actively contract the antagonist, or opposing muscle group.
3. Move into the stretch quickly and smoothly.
4. Hold for 1 to 2 seconds and then release the stretch.
5. Repeat 5 to 10 times.

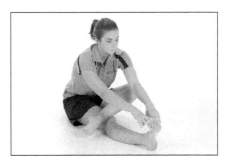

While AI stretching certainly has some benefits (mainly for the professional or well conditioned athlete), it also has a number of unsubstantiated claims. One such claim is that AI stretching does not engage the stretch reflex (or myotatic reflex) because the stretch is only held for 2 seconds or less.[1,2] This however, defies basic muscle physiology. The stretch reflex in the calf muscle for example is triggered within 3 hundredths of a second, so any claim that AI stretching can somehow bypass or outsmart the stretch reflex is nothing more than wishful thinking.

Resistance Stretching and Loaded Stretching

Resistance stretching and loaded stretching are a form of dynamic stretching that both contract and lengthen a muscle at the same time. They work by stretching a muscle group through its entire range of motion while under contraction. For this reason, both resistance stretching and loaded stretching are as much about strengthening a muscle group as they are about stretching it.

Like AI stretching above, resistance stretching and loaded stretching do have their benefits. Five time Olympic swimmer, Dara Torres credits a portion of her swimming success to the use of resistance stretching. However, these forms of stretching place high demands on the musculo-skeletal system and are therefore only recommended for professional or well conditioned athletes.

---

[1] Mattes, A. 2000 *Active Isolated Stretching: The Mattes Method* Pages 1, 3, 6.
[2] Wharton, J & P. 1996 *The Whartons' Stretch Book* Page xxiii.

Chapter 5
The Rules for Safe Stretching

As with most activities there are rules and guidelines to ensure that they are safe. Stretching is no exception. Stretching can be extremely dangerous and harmful if done incorrectly. It is vitally important that the following rules be adhered to, both for safety and for maximizing the potential benefits of stretching.

There is often confusion and concerns about which stretches are good and which stretches are bad. In most cases someone has told the inquirer that they should not do this stretch or that stretch, or that this is a "good" stretch and this is a "bad" stretch.

Are there only good stretches and bad stretches? Is there no middle ground? And if there are only good and bad stretches, how do we decide which ones are good and which ones are bad? Let us put an end to the confusion once and for all.

There is no such thing as a good or bad stretch!

Just as there are no good or bad exercises, there are no good or bad stretches; only what is appropriate for the specific requirements of the individual. So a stretch that is perfectly safe and beneficial for one person may not be safe or beneficial for someone else.

Let us use an example. A person with a shoulder injury would not be expected to do push-ups or freestyle swimming, but that does not mean that these are bad exercises. Now, consider the same scenario from a stretching point of view. That same person should avoid shoulder stretches, but that does not mean that all shoulder stretches are bad.

The stretch itself is neither good nor bad. It is the way the stretch is performed and whom it is performed on that makes stretching either effective and safe, or ineffective and harmful. To place a particular stretch into the category of "good" or "bad" is foolish and dangerous. To label a stretch as "good" gives people the false impression that they can do that stretch whenever and however they want and it will not cause them any harm or injury, which is misleading and dangerous.

The specific requirements of the individual are what are important!

Remember, stretches are neither good nor bad. However, when choosing a stretch there are a number of precautions and checks that need to be performed before giving that stretch the okay.

1. **Firstly, make a general review of the individual.** Are they healthy and physically active, or have they been leading a sedentary lifestyle for the past 5 years? Are they a professional athlete? Are they recovering from a serious injury? Do they have aches, pains or muscle and joint stiffness in any area of their body?

2. **Secondly, make a specific review of the area, or muscle group to be stretched.** Are the muscles healthy? Is there any damage to the joints, ligaments, tendons, etc.? Has the area been injured recently, or is it still recovering from an injury?

If the muscle group being stretched is not 100% healthy, avoid stretching that area altogether. Work on recovery and rehabilitation before moving onto specific stretching exercises. If however, the individual is healthy and the area to be stretched is free from injury, then apply the following rules and guidelines to all stretches.

Warm-up prior to stretching

This first rule is often overlooked and can lead to serious injury if not performed effectively. Trying to stretch muscles that have not been warmed, is like trying to stretch old, dry rubber bands; they may snap.

Warming up prior to stretching does a number of beneficial things, but primarily its purpose is to prepare the body and mind for more strenuous activity. One of the ways it achieves this is by increasing the body's core temperature while also increasing the body's muscle temperature. This helps to make the muscles loose, supple and pliable, and is essential to ensure the maximum benefits are gained from stretching.

A correct warm-up also has the effect of increasing both heart rate and respiratory rate. This increases blood flow, which in turn increases the delivery of oxygen and nutrients to the working muscles. All this helps to prepare the muscles for stretching.

A correct warm-up should consist of light physical activity, like walking, jogging or easy aerobics. Both the intensity and duration of the warm-up (or how hard and how long), should be governed by the fitness level of the participating athlete, although a correct warm-up for most people should take about five to ten minutes and result in a light sweat.

For more information about stretching and the warm-up, refer to *How to use Stretching as part of the Warm-up* in chapter 6.

Stretch before and after exercise

The question often arises: *Should I stretch before or after exercise?* This is not an either / or situation; both are essential. It is no good stretching after exercise and counting that as the pre-exercise stretch for next time. Stretching after exercise has a totally different purpose to stretching before exercise.

The purpose of stretching before exercise is to prepare the individual for activity and help prevent injury. Stretching does this by lengthening the muscles and associated soft tissues, which in turn increases range of motion. This ensures that we are able to move freely without restriction or injury occurring.

However, stretching after exercise has a very different role. Its purpose is primarily to aid in the repair and recovery of the muscles and associated soft tissues. By lengthening the muscles, stretching helps to prevent tight muscles and delayed onset muscle soreness (DOMS) that sometimes accompanies strenuous exercise.

After exercise stretching should be done as part of a cool-down. The cool-down will vary depending on the duration and intensity of exercise undertaken, but will usually consist of five to ten minutes of very light physical activity and be followed by five to ten minutes of static stretching exercises.

An effective cool-down involving light physical activity and stretching will help to: rid waste products from the muscles; prevent blood pooling; and promote the delivery of oxygen and nutrients to the muscles. All this helps to return the body to a pre-exercise level, thus aiding the recovery process.

Stretch all major muscles and their opposing muscle groups

When stretching, it is vitally important that attention is paid to all the major muscle groups in the body. Just because a particular sport places a lot of emphasis on the legs, for example, does not mean that one can neglect the muscles of the upper body in a stretching routine.

All the muscles play an important role in any physical activity, not just a select few. Muscles in the upper body, for example, are extremely important in any running sport. They play a vital role in the stability and balance of the body during the running motion. Therefore it is important to keep them both flexible and supple.

Every muscle in the body has an opposing muscle that acts against it. For example, the muscles in the front of the leg, (the quadriceps) are opposed by the muscles in the back of the leg, (the hamstrings). These two groups of muscles provide a resistance to each other that balance the body. If one group of muscles becomes stronger or more flexible than the other group, it is likely to lead to imbalances that can result in injury or postural problems.

For example, hamstring tears are a common injury in most running sports. They are often caused by strong quadriceps and weak, inflexible hamstrings. This imbalance puts a great deal of pressure on the hamstrings and can result in a muscle tear or strain.

The same principle applies to the left and right sides of the body. Some sports and activities place more emphasis on one side of the body, which can result in differing levels of flexibility from one side of the body to the other.

For example, baseball pitchers often develop an imbalance between their pitching arm and their non pitching arm. Typically the pitching arm and shoulder become stronger and tighter than the non pitching arm and shoulder. This can lead to uneven forces that pull on the cervical and thoracic regions of the spine, resulting in abnormal curvature, which can increase the likelihood of injuries to the neck, upper back and shoulders.

Stretch gently and slowly
Stretching gently and slowly helps to relax the muscles, which in turn makes stretching more pleasurable and beneficial. This will also help to avoid muscle tears and strains that can be caused by rapid, jerky movements.

Stretch ONLY to the point of tension
Stretching is NOT an activity that is meant to be painful; it should be pleasurable, relaxing and very beneficial. Although many people believe that to get the most from their stretching they need to be in constant pain. This is one of the greatest mistakes that can be made when stretching. Let me explain why.

When the muscles are stretched to the point of pain, the body employs a defense mechanism called the *stretch reflex* (or myotatic reflex). This is the body's safety measure to prevent serious damage occurring to the muscles, tendons and joints. The stretch reflex protects the muscles and tendons by contracting them, thereby preventing them from being stretched.

So to avoid the stretch reflex, avoid pain. Never push the stretch beyond what is comfortable. Only stretch to the point where tension can be felt in the muscles. This way, injury will be avoided and the maximum benefits from stretching will be achieved.

Breathe slowly and easily while stretching

Many people unconsciously hold their breath while stretching. This causes tension in the muscles, which in turn makes it very difficult to stretch. To avoid this, remember to breathe slowly and deeply during all stretching exercises. This helps to relax the muscles, promotes blood flow and increases the delivery of oxygen and nutrients to the muscles.

An example

By taking a look at one of the most controversial stretches ever performed, we can see how the above rules are applied.

The stretch below causes a negative response from many people. It has a reputation as a dangerous, bad stretch and should be avoided at all costs.

So why is it that at every Olympic Games, Commonwealth Games and World Championships, sprinters can be seen doing this stretch before their events? Let us apply the above checks to find out.

Firstly, consider the person performing the stretch. Are they healthy, fit and physically active? If not, this is not a stretch they should be doing. Are they elderly, overweight or unfit? Are they young and still growing? Do they lead a sedentary lifestyle? If so, they should avoid this stretch.

This first consideration alone would most likely prohibit 25% of the population from doing this stretch.

Secondly, review the area to be stretched. This stretch obviously places a large strain on the muscles of the hamstrings and lower back, so if the hamstrings or lower back are not 100% healthy, do not do this stretch.

With the high occurrence of back pain among the population, this second consideration could easily rule out another 50%, which means this stretch is only suitable for about 25% of the population. Or, the well trained, physically fit, injury free athlete. Then apply the six precautions above and the well trained, physically fit, injury free athlete can perform this stretch safely and effectively.

Remember, the stretch itself is neither good, nor bad. It is the way the stretch is performed and whom it is performed on that makes stretching either effective and safe, or ineffective and harmful.

Chapter 6
How to Stretch Properly

When to stretch?

Stretching needs to be as important as the rest of our training. If we are involved in any competitive type of sport or exercise then it is crucial that we make time for specific stretching workouts. Set time aside to work on muscle groups that are tight or especially important for your particular sport. The more involved and committed we are to exercise and fitness, the more time and effort we will need to commit to stretching.

As discussed in chapter 5 it is important to stretch both before and after exercise, but when else should we stretch? Stretch periodically throughout the entire day. It is a great way to stay loose and to help ease the stress of everyday life. One of the most productive ways to utilize time is to stretch while watching television. Start with five minutes of marching or jogging on the spot then take a seat on the floor in front of the television and start stretching.

Competition is a time when great demands are placed on the body; therefore it is vitally important that we are in peak physical condition. Flexibility should be at its best just before competition. Too many injuries are caused by the sudden exertion that is needed for competitive sport. Get strict on stretching before competition.

What type of stretching?

Choosing the right type of stretching for the right purpose will make a big difference to the effectiveness of any flexibility training program. To follow are some suggestions for when to use the different types of stretches. (For more detailed information refer to chapter 4.)

For warming up, dynamic stretching is the most effective, while for cooling down, static, passive and PNF stretching are best. For improving range of motion, try PNF and Active Isolated stretching, and for injury rehabilitation, a combination of PNF, Isometric and Active stretching will give the best results.

Hold, Count, Repeat

For how long should we hold each stretch? How often should we stretch? For how long should we stretch?

These are the most commonly asked questions when discussing the topic of stretching. Although there are conflicting responses to these questions, it is my professional opinion, that through a study of research literature and personal experience, I believe what follows is currently the most correct and beneficial information.

The question that causes the most conflict is: *For how long should I hold each stretch?* For Static and Passive stretching, some text will say that as little as ten seconds is enough. This is a bare minimum. Ten seconds is only just enough time for the muscles to relax and start to lengthen. For any real improvement to flexibility, each stretch should be held for at least twenty to thirty seconds.

The time committed to stretching should be relative to the level of involvement in our particular sport. So, for people looking to increase their general level of health and fitness, a minimum of about twenty seconds will be enough. However, if involved in high level competitive sport we need to hold each stretch for at least thirty seconds and start to extend that to sixty seconds and beyond.

How often should I stretch? The same principle of adjusting the level of commitment to the level of involvement in our sport applies to the number of times we should stretch each muscle group. For example, the beginner should stretch each muscle group two to three times. However, if involved at a more advanced level, we should stretch each muscle group three to five times.

For how long should I stretch? The same principle applies. For the beginner, about five to ten minutes is enough, and for the professional athlete, anything up to two hours. If we are somewhere between the beginner and professional adjust the time spent stretching accordingly.

Do not be impatient with stretching. Nobody can get fit in a couple of weeks, so do not expect miracles from a stretching routine. Looking long term, some muscle groups may need a minimum of three months of regular stretching to see any real improvement. So stick with it, it is well worth the effort.

Sequence
When starting a stretching program it is a good idea to start with a general range of stretches for the entire body, instead of just a select few. The idea of this is to reduce overall muscle tension and to increase the mobility of the joints and limbs.

The next step should be to increase overall flexibility by starting to extend the muscles beyond their normal range of motion. Following this; work on specific areas that are tight or important for your particular sport. Remember, all this takes time. This sequence of stretches may take up to three months to see real improvement, especially if we have no background in agility based activities or are heavily muscled.

Limited data exists on what order individual stretches should be done in. However, some researchers have suggested designing flexibility training programs that start with the core muscles of the stomach, sides, back and neck, and then work out to the extremities. Others have recommended starting with sitting stretches, because there is less chance of accidental injury while sitting, before moving on to standing stretches.

The exact order in which individual stretches are done is not the main point of emphasis; the main priority is to cover all the major muscle groups and their opposing muscles, and to work on those areas that are most tight or more important for your specific sport.

Once we have advanced beyond improving overall flexibility and are working on improving the range of motion of specific muscles, or muscle groups, it is important to isolate those muscles during the stretching routines. To do this, concentrate on only one muscle group at a time. For example, instead of trying to stretch both hamstrings at the same time, concentrate on only one at a time. Stretching this way will help to reduce the resistance from other supporting muscle groups.

Posture

Posture, or alignment, while stretching is one of the most neglected aspects of flexibility training. It is important to be aware of how crucial it can be to the overall benefits of stretching. Poor posture and incorrect alignment can cause imbalances in the muscles that can lead to injury. While proper posture will ensure that the targeted muscle group receives the best possible stretch.

In many instances one major muscle group can be made up of a number of different muscles. If posture is poor or incorrect certain stretching exercises may put more emphasis on one particular muscle within that muscle group, thus causing an imbalance that could lead to injury.

The picture on the right, for example, shows the difference between good posture and poor posture when stretching the hamstring muscles (the muscles at the back of the upper legs).

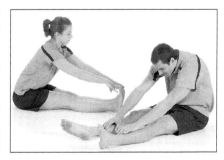

During this stretch it is important to keep both feet pointing straight up. Allowing the feet to fall to one side will put more emphasis on one particular part of the hamstrings, which could result in a muscle imbalance.

Note the athlete on the left; feet upright and back relatively straight. The athlete on the right is at a greater risk of causing a muscular imbalance that may lead to injury.

How to use stretching as part of the warm-up

Lately, I have been receiving a lot of questions referring to recent studies and research findings about stretching. The most common question I receive concerns the role that stretching plays as part of the warm-up procedure.

Currently, there seems to be a lot of confusion about how and when stretching should be used as part of the warm-up, and some people are under the impression that stretching should be avoided altogether.

This is a very important issue and needs to be clarified immediately. The following information is provided to dispel some common myths and misconceptions about stretching and its role as part of the warm-up.

What has science got to say?

Most of the studies I have reviewed attempt to determine the short term, or one-off effects of stretching on injury prevention. This is a mistake in itself and shows a lack of understanding as to how stretching is used as part of a conditioning or injury prevention program.

Stretching and its effect on physical performance and injury prevention is something that just cannot be measured scientifically. Sure we can measure the effect of stretching on flexibility with simple tests like the *Sit and Reach Test*, but then to determine how that effects athletic performance or injury susceptibility is very difficult, if not near impossible. One of the more recent studies on stretching supports this view by concluding; *Due to the paucity, heterogeneity and poor quality of the available studies no definitive conclusions can be drawn as to the value of stretching for reducing the risk of exercise-related injury.*[1]

To put the above quote in layman's terms; there has not been enough studies done and the studies that have been done are not specific or consistent enough.

---

[1] Weldon, SM. The efficacy of stretching for prevention of exercise-related injury: a systematic review of the literature. *Manual Therapy*, 2003 Volume 8, Issue 3, Page 141.

The greatest misconception

Confusion about what stretching accomplishes, as part of the warm-up procedure, is causing many to abandon stretching altogether. The key to understanding the role stretching plays can be found in the previous sentence; but you have to read it carefully.

Stretching, as part of the warm-up!

Here is the key: Stretching is a critical part of the warm-up, but stretching is NOT the warm-up.

Do not make the mistake of thinking that doing a few stretches constitutes a warm-up. An effective warm-up has a number of very important key elements, which all work together to minimize the likelihood of sports injury and prepare the individual for physical activity.

Identifying the components of an effective and safe warm-up, and executing them in the correct order is critical. Remember, stretching is only one part of an effective warm-up, and its place in the warm-up procedure is specific and dependant on the other components.

The four key elements that should be included to ensure an effective and complete warm-up are:

1. **The general warm-up**: This phase of the warm-up consists of 5 to 15 minutes of light physical activity. The aim here is to elevate the heart rate and respiratory rate, increase blood flow and increase muscle temperature.

2. **Static stretching**: Next, a few minutes of gentle static stretching should be incorporated into the general warm-up to gradually lengthen all the major muscle groups and associated soft tissues of the body.

3. **The sports specific warm-up**: During this phase of the warm-up, 10 to 15 minutes of sport specific drills and exercises should be used to prepare the athlete for the specific demands of their chosen sport.

4. **Dynamic stretching**: Lastly, the warm-up procedure should finish with a number of dynamic stretching exercises that mimic the common movements of the sport or activity to follow. For example, arm rotations for swimming, or swing kicks for running sports. Remember, the force of the bounce or swing is gradually increased but should never become radical or uncontrolled.

All four parts are equally important and any one part should not be neglected or thought of as not necessary. All four elements work together to bring the body and mind to a physical peak, ensuring the athlete is prepared for the activity to come.

Please note the following points

1. Dynamic stretching carries with it an increased risk of injury if used incorrectly. Refer to chapter 4 for more information about dynamic stretching.

2. The time recommendations given in the above warm-up procedure relate specifically to the requirements of a serious athlete. Adjust the times accordingly if your athletic participation is not of a professional manner.

3. Recent studies have indicated that static stretching may have a negative effect on muscle contraction speed and therefore impair performance of athletes involved in sports requiring high levels of power and speed. It is for this reason that static stretching is conducted early in the warm-up procedure and is always followed by sports specific drills and dynamic stretching. Recent studies suggest no detrimental effects when static stretching is conducted early in the warm-up.[2]

What conclusions can we make?

Stretching is beneficial, when used correctly. Remember, stretching is just one important component that assists to reduce the risk of injury and improve athletic performance. The best results are achieved when stretching is used in combination with other injury reduction techniques and conditioning exercises.

---

[2] Taylor, KL. Sheppard, JM. Lee, H. Plummer, N. Negative effect of static stretching restored when combined with a sports specific warm-up component. *Journal of Science and Medicine in Sport*, 2009 Nov; 12(6):657-61.

Chapter 7
Flexibility Testing

To really take advantage of the many benefits of stretching, a record of flexibility should be kept. For sports trainers and coaches in particular, it is vitally important to test and chart an athletes' flexibility on a regular basis. This is important for two reasons.

Firstly, it provides a starting point from which to measure improvements and gives an indication of any areas that may be weak, limited or inflexible.

Secondly, in the event of an injury, this baseline flexibility provides a goal to achieve before resuming exercise or returning to competition. It is vitally important that flexibility is regained after an injury. Therefore having a record of what the level of flexibility was before the injury is very useful as a target to achieve.

During the year set a minimum standard of flexibility for the activities engaged in. If an athlete becomes injured, it should be the goal to achieve the minimum standard of flexibility required for that activity before returning to exercise, competition or strenuous training.

What follows is a brief example of a few basic flexibility tests. These are the most commonly used tests but they are by no means the only ones. If more are required, consult a professional sports trainer for ideas about tests that are specific to the athletes' particular sport. Remember *The Rules for Safe Stretching* in chapter 5 and once a test is used it is important not to vary it in any way. It must be kept the same each time it is used.

All the following tests are best done using a goniometer; a devise for measuring body limb angles. If a goniometer is not available, any standard 360 degree protractor will give a good indication of the angle at a particular joint.

Sit and Reach Test
The sit and reach test is probably the most common test used to measure flexibility in the back, hips and hamstring muscles.

Sit on the floor with your legs straight and your feet flat

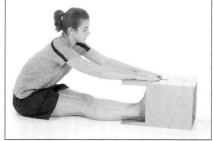

against an upright board. Bend forward reaching towards, or as far past, your toes as possible, and then record the distance reached. This test will give a good indication of hamstring, hip and back flexibility.

Shoulder Flexibility Test

Unfortunately, participants in sports such as swimming, tennis (or any racket sport), any of the throwing events in athletics and especially contact sports, are extremely susceptible to injuries of the shoulder. Shoulder flexibility should be a prime concern for anyone participating in these sports.

Start by standing upright with the hand pointing down. In this position the hand represents the 0 degree position.

Then raise the arm directly forward and above the head, as in the picture to the right. Its furthest point is then recorded. An average acceptable reading of 180 degrees is expected for athletes.

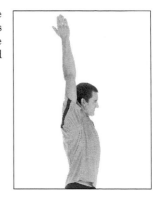

Now move the arm down and behind the back to its furthest position, as in the picture to the right. This measurement is recorded and should exceed 50 degrees.

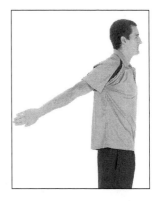

Hamstring Flexibility Test

Lie on the ground face up, with arms straight beside the body, as in the picture below. Raise one leg as far up as possible. Keep the leg straight and measure the angle at the hip joint. An angle of 90 degrees is considered average to good.

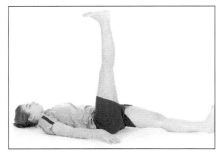

Chapter 8
135 Unique Stretching Exercises

In this second half of the book there are 135 photographs of unique stretching exercises, each with an accompanying description explaining how the stretch is performed. These stretching exercises are not specific to any particular sport or any particular type of person. Of course all of them will not be relevant to everyone, but a great number of them will be suitable for most athletes, coaches, trainers and health care professionals.

If you find a particular stretch difficult to perform, start with the stretches that are more comfortable for you, and return to the more difficult stretches when your flexibility has improved.

An index is included on page 44 to assist in finding individual stretches, and each stretch has been arranged to correspond with a particular body part or major muscle group. For example, when looking for stretches for the shoulders, look to that particular heading. The stretches have been arranged so as to start with the neck and work down to the ankles and feet.

On the following two pages there are anatomical diagrams of the major muscles of the body, and at the beginning of each section there is a list of the individual muscles that the stretches target. By matching the list of individual muscles at the beginning of each section, with the anatomical diagrams on the next two pages, you can see exactly which muscles are being stretched during each stretching exercise.

For a more comprehensive explanation of the muscle anatomy involved during each of the stretching exercises, please refer to *The Anatomy of Stretching* at www.AnatomyOfStretching.com.

Important!
Remember to always follow *The Rules for Safe Stretching* in chapter 5, and if you have any pre-existing injuries or ailments please consult a sports doctor or physical therapist before attempting any of the following stretches. Discontinue any exercise that causes pain or severe discomfort and consult a medical expert.

Muscular System (anterior view)

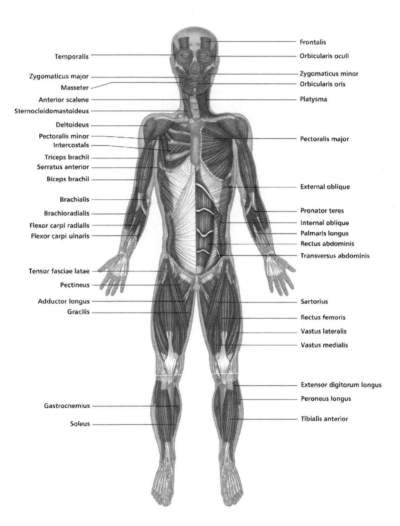

135 Unique Stretching Exercises

Muscular System (posterior view)

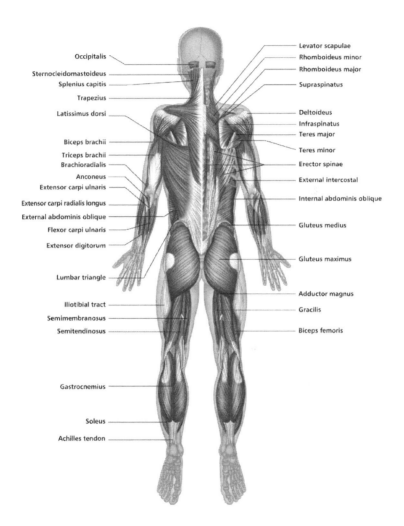

Copyright © 2003 Chris Jarmey - The Concise Book of Muscles
www.MuscleAnatomyPictures.com

Index of Stretches

A.	Neck and Shoulders (17)	45
B.	Arms and Chest (17)	55
C.	Stomach (6)	65
D.	Back and Sides (23)	69
E.	Hips and Buttocks (13)	83
F.	Quadriceps (7)	91
G.	Hamstrings (15)	97
H.	Adductors (8)	107
I.	Abductors (7)	113
J.	Upper Calves (8)	119
K.	Lower Calves and Achilles (8)	125
L.	Shins, Ankles, Feet and Toes (6)	131

Stretches for the Neck and Shoulders

The neck and shoulders are comprised of a multitude of small muscles that control the head and upper arm. The muscles around the neck and shoulder, along with the structure of the joints, allow for a large range of motion of the head and upper arm; including flexion, extension, adduction, abduction and rotation.

The anatomical structures of the neck and shoulder joints are commonly over-stretched by applying too much force to the targeted muscle groups. Please take extra care when performing the following stretches and always follow *The Rules for Safe Stretching* in chapter 5.

Sports that benefit from these neck and shoulder stretches include: Archery; batting sports like Cricket, Baseball and Softball; Boxing; contact sports like Football, Gridiron and Rugby; Golf; racquet sports like Tennis, Badminton and Squash; Swimming; throwing sports like Cricket, Baseball and Field events; and Wrestling.

The major muscles being stretched.

Deltoid anterior, medius, posterior
Infraspinatus
Levator scapulae
Longissimus capitis
Longissimus cervicis
Omohyoid
Platysma
Scalenus anterior, medius,
posterior
Semispinalis capitis
Semispinalis cervicis
Serratus anterior

Spinalis capitis
Spinalis cervicis
Splenius capitis
Splenius cervicis
Sternocleidomastoid
Sternohyoid
Sternothyroid
Subscapularis
Supraspinatus
Teres major
Teres minor
Trapezius

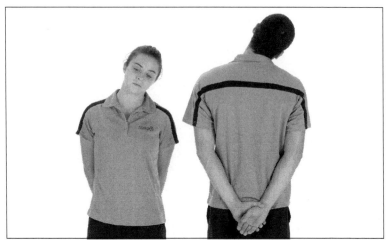

A01 - Lateral Neck Stretch: Look forward while keeping your head up. Slowly move your ear towards your shoulder while keeping your hands behind your back.

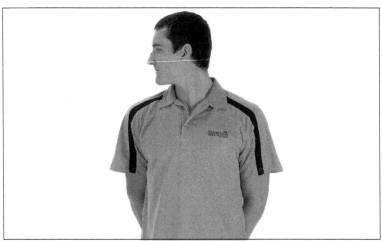

A02 - Rotating Neck Stretch: Stand upright while keeping your shoulders still and your head up, then slowly rotate your chin towards your shoulder.

Stretches for the Neck and Shoulders

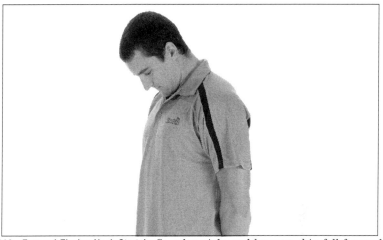

A03 - Forward Flexion Neck Stretch: Stand upright and let your chin fall forward towards your chest. Relax your shoulders and keep your hands by your side.

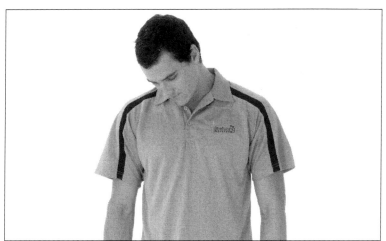

A04 - Diagonal Flexion Neck Stretch: Stand upright and let your chin fall forward towards your chest. Then gently lean your head to one side.

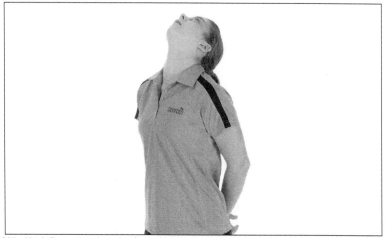

A05 - Neck Extension Stretch: Stand upright and lift your head, looking upwards as if trying to point up with your chin. Relax your shoulders and keep your hands by your side.

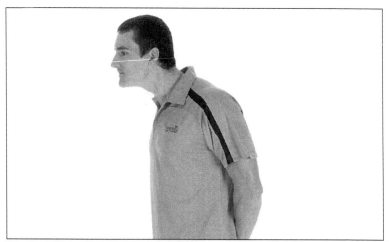

A06 - Neck Protraction Stretch: While looking straight ahead, push your head forward by sticking your chin out.

Stretches for the Neck and Shoulders

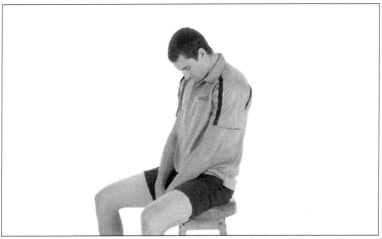

A07 - Sitting Neck Flexion Stretch: While sitting on a chair, cross your arms and hold onto the chair between your legs. Let your head fall forward and then lean backwards.

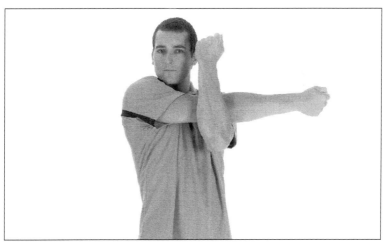

A08 - Parallel Arm Shoulder Stretch: Stand upright and place one arm across your body. Keep your arm parallel to the ground and pull your elbow towards your body.

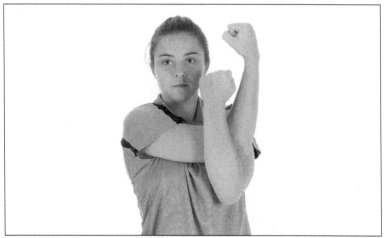

A09 - Bent Arm Shoulder Stretch: Stand upright and place one arm across your body. Bend your arm at 90 degrees and pull your elbow towards your body.

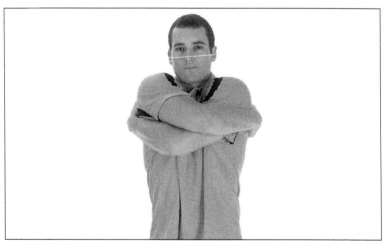

A10 - Wrap-around Shoulder Stretch: Stand upright and wrap your arms around your shoulders as if hugging yourself. Pull your shoulders back.

Stretches for the Neck and Shoulders

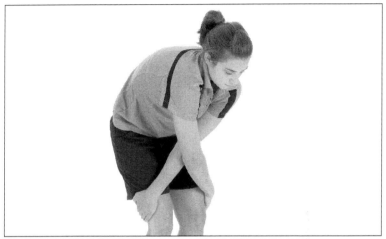

A11 - Cross-over Shoulder Stretch: Stand with your knees bent. Cross your arms over and grab the back of your knees, then start to rise upwards until you feel tension in your upper back and shoulders.

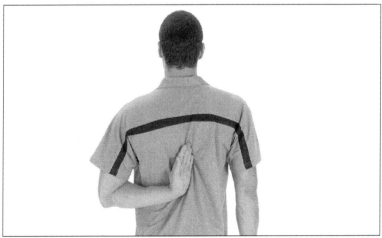

A12 - Reaching-up Shoulder Stretch: Place one hand behind your back and then reach up between your shoulder blades.

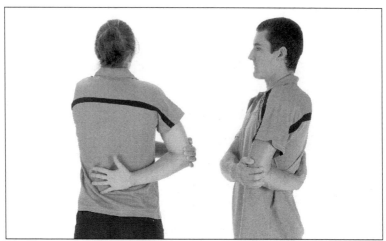

A13 - Elbow-out Rotator Stretch: Stand with your hand behind the middle of your back and your elbow pointing out. Reach over with your other hand and gently pull your elbow forward.

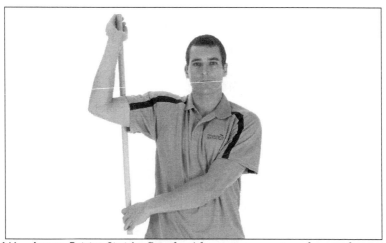

A14 - Arm-up Rotator Stretch: Stand with your arm out and your forearm pointing upwards at 90 degrees. Place a broom stick in your hand and behind your elbow. With your other hand pull the bottom of the broom stick forward.

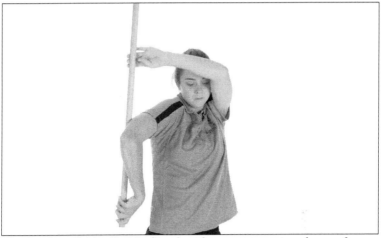

A15 - Arm-down Rotator Stretch: Stand with your arm out and your forearm pointing downwards at 90 degrees. Place a broom stick in your hand and behind your elbow. With your other hand pull the top of the broom stick forward.

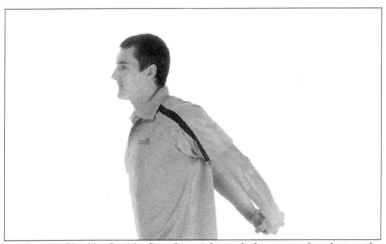

A16 - Reverse Shoulder Stretch: Stand upright and clasp your hands together behind your back. Keep your arms straight and slowly lift your hands upward.

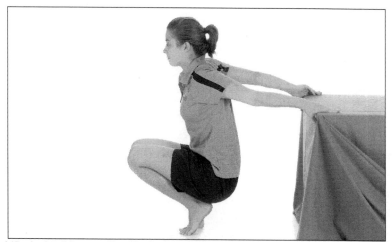

A17 - Assisted Reverse Shoulder Stretch: Stand upright with your back towards a table or bench and place your hands on the edge of the table or bench. Keep your arms straight and slowly lower your entire body.

Stretches for the Arms and Chest

The arms and chest are comprised of a number of both large muscles (Pectoralis major, biceps) and small muscles (Pectoarlis minor, teres major). These muscles are primarily responsible for shoulder stabilization and arm movement.

Sports that benefit from these arm and chest stretches include: Archery; Basketball and Netball; batting sports like Cricket, Baseball and Softball; Hiking, Backpacking, Mountaineering and Orienteering; Ice hockey and Field hockey; Martial Arts; racquet sports like Tennis, Badminton and Squash; Rowing, Canoeing and Kayaking; Swimming; throwing sports like Cricket, Baseball and Field events; Volleyball; and Wrestling.

The major muscles being stretched.
Biceps brachii
Brachialis
Brachioradialis
Coracobrachialis
Extensor carpi radialis longus and brevis
Extensor carpi ulnaris
Extensor digiti minimi
Extensor digitorum
Extensor indicis
Extensor pollicis longus and brevis
Flexor carpi radialis
Flexor carpi ulnaris
Flexor digitorum profundus
Flexor digitorum superficialis
Flexor pollicus brevis
Flexor pollicis longus
Opponens digiti minimi
Opponens pollicis
Palmer interossei
Palmaris longus
Pectoralis major
Pectorilis minor
Pronator teres
Supinator
Triceps

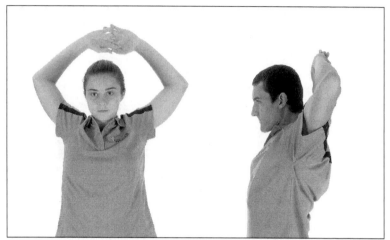

B01 - Above Head Chest Stretch: Stand upright and interlock your fingers. Bend your arms and place them above your head while forcing your elbows and hands backwards.

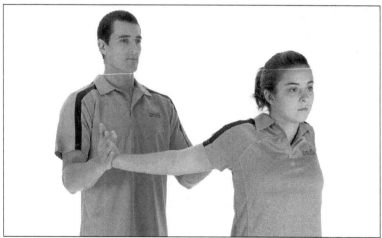

B02 - Partner Assisted Chest Stretch: Extend both arms parallel to the ground and have a partner hold on to your hands, then slowly pull your arms backwards.

Stretches for the Arms and Chest

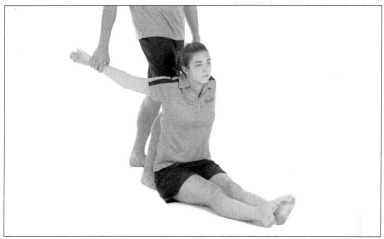

B03 - Seated Partner Assisted Chest Stretch: Sit on the ground and have a partner stand behind you. Reach behind with both arms and have the partner further extend your arms.

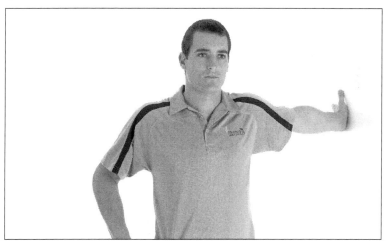

B04 - Parallel Arm Chest Stretch: Stand with your arm extended to the rear and parallel to the ground. Hold on to an immovable object and then turn your shoulders and body away from your outstretched arm.

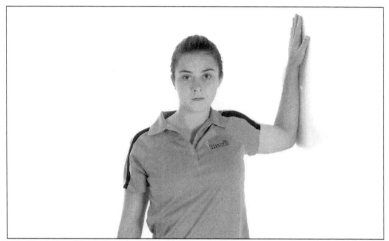

B05 - Bent Arm Chest Stretch: Stand with your arm extended and your forearm pointing up at 90 degrees. Rest your forearm against an immovable object and then turn your shoulders and body away from your extended arm.

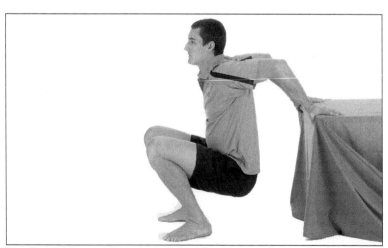

B06 - Assisted Reverse Chest Stretch: Stand upright with your back towards a table or bench and place your hands on the edge of the table or bench. Bend your arms and slowly lower your entire body.

Stretches for the Arms and Chest

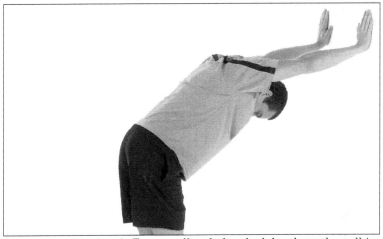

B07 - Bent-over Chest Stretch: Face a wall and place both hands on the wall just above your head. Slowly lower your shoulders as if moving your chin towards the ground.

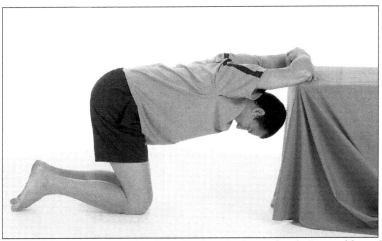

B08 - Kneeling Chest Stretch: Kneel on the floor in front of a chair or table and interlock your forearms above your head. Place your arms on the object and lower your upper body toward the ground.

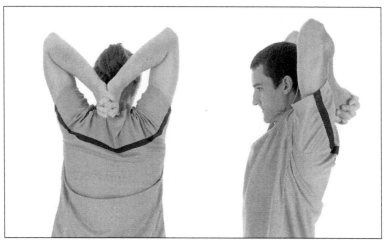

B09 - Reaching-down Triceps Stretch: Reach behind your head with both hands and your elbows pointing upwards. Then reach down your back with your hands.

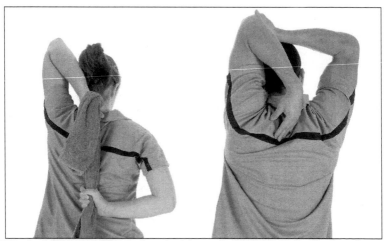

B10 - Assisted Triceps Stretch: Stand with one hand behind your neck and your elbow pointing upwards. Then use your other hand (or a rope or towel) to pull your elbow down.

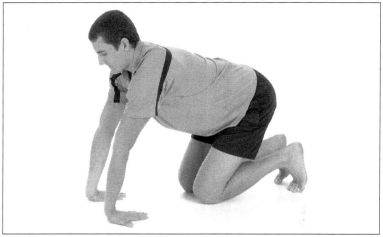

B11 - Kneeling Forearm Stretch: While crouching on your knees with your forearms facing forward and hands pointing backwards, slowly move rearward.

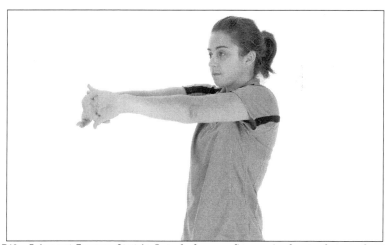

B12 - Palms-out Forearm Stretch: Interlock your fingers in front of your chest, then straighten your arms and turn the palms of your hands so that they face outwards.

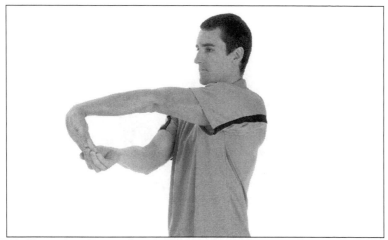

B13 - Fingers-down Forearm Stretch: Hold onto your fingers and turn your palms outwards. Straighten your arm and then pull your fingers back using your other hand.

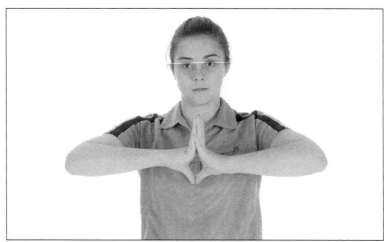

B14 - Finger Stretch: Place the tips of your fingers together and push your palms towards each other.

Stretches for the Arms and Chest

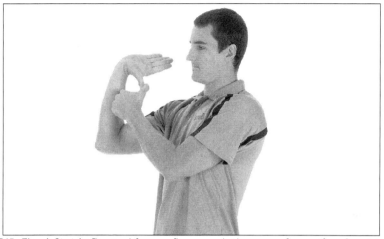

B15 - Thumb Stretch: Start with your fingers pointing up and your thumb out to one side, then use your other hand to pull your thumb down.

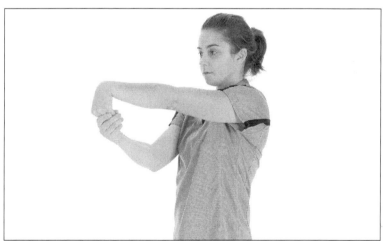

B16 - Fingers-down Wrist Stretch: Hold on to your fingers and straighten your arm, then pull your fingers towards your body.

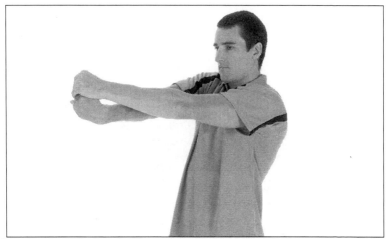

B17 - Rotating Wrist Stretch: Place one arm straight out in front and parallel to the ground. Rotate your wrist down and outwards and then use your other hand to further rotate your hand upwards.

Stretches for the Stomach

The muscles around the stomach extend from the bottom of the rib cage down to the front of the pelvic bone. The primary action of the stomach muscles is to both flex and rotate the lumbar spine.

Sports that benefit from these stomach stretches include: Basketball and Netball; batting sports like Cricket, Baseball and Softball; Boxing; contact sports like Football, Gridiron and Rugby; Golf; Hiking, Backpacking, Mountaineering and Orienteering; Ice Hockey and Field Hockey; Ice Skating, Roller Skating and Inline Skating; Martial Arts; Rowing, Canoeing and Kayaking; Running, Track and Cross Country; running sports like Football, Soccer, Gridiron and Rugby; Snow Skiing and Water Skiing; Surfing; Walking and Race Walking; and Wrestling.

The major muscles being stretched.
Obliques external and internal
Transversus abdominis
Rectus abdominis

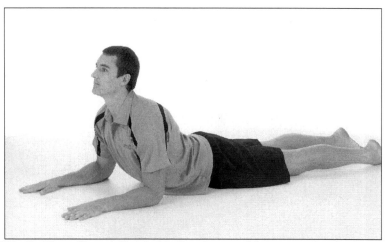

C01 - On Elbows Stomach Stretch: Lie face down and bring your hands close to your shoulders. Keep your hips on the ground, look forward and rise up onto your elbows.

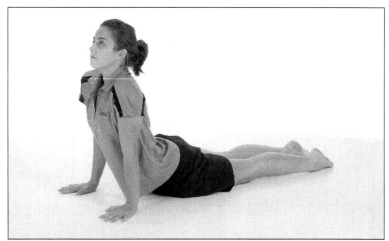

C02 - Rising Stomach Stretch: Lie face down and bring your hands close to your shoulders. Keep your hips on the ground, look forward and rise up by straightening your arms.

Stretches for the Stomach

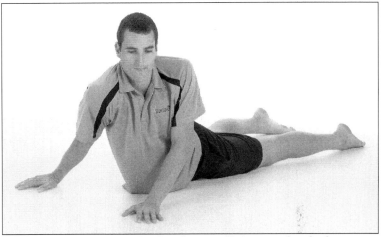

C03 - Rotating Stomach Stretch: Lie face down and bring your hands close to your shoulders. Keep your hips on the ground, look forward and rise up by straightening your arms. Then slowly bend one arm and rotate that shoulder towards the ground.

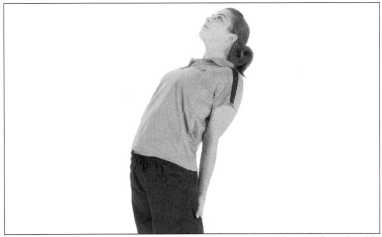

C04 - Standing Lean-back Stomach Stretch: Stand upright with your feet shoulder width apart and place your hands on your buttocks for support. Look upwards and slowly lean backwards at the waist.

67

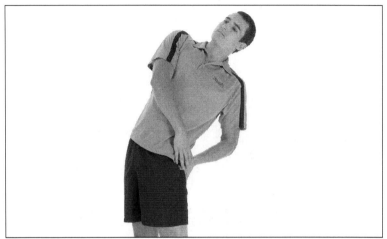

C05 - Standing Lean-back Side Stomach Stretch: Stand upright with your feet shoulder width apart and place one hand of your buttocks. Look up and slowly lean backwards at the waist, then reach over with your opposite hand and rotate at the waist.

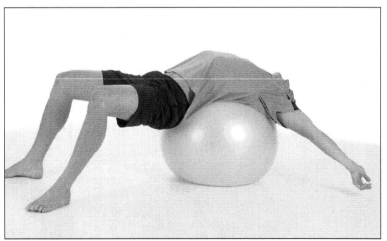

C06 - Back Arching Stomach Stretch: Sit on a Swiss ball and slowly roll the ball forward while leaning back. Allow your back and shoulders to rest on the ball and your arms to hang to each side.

Stretches for the Back and Sides

The muscles around the spine, and the broader area of the back, are primarily responsible for stabilizing the spinal column and keeping the back in an upright position. The muscles of the back and sides allow the upper body and spine to move in flexion, extension and rotation.

Sports that benefit from these back and side stretches include: Archery; Basketball and Netball; batting sports like Cricket, Baseball and Softball; Boxing; contact sports like Football, Rugby and Gridiron; Cycling; Golf; Hiking, Backpacking, Mountaineering and Orienteering; Ice Hockey and Field Hockey; Ice Skating, Roller Skating and Inline Skating; Martial Arts; racquet sports like Tennis, Badminton and Squash; Rowing, Canoeing and Kayaking; Running, Track and Cross Country; running sports like Football, Soccer, Gridiron and Rugby; Snow Skiing and Water Skiing; Surfing; Swimming; throwing sports like Cricket, Baseball and Field events; Volleyball; Walking and Race Walking; and Wrestling.

The major muscles being stretched.

Iliocostalis cervicis
Iliocostalis thoracis
Iliocostalis lumborum
Intercostals external and internal
Interspinales
Intertransversarii
Latissimus dorsi
Longissimus thoracis
Multifidus
Quadratus lumborum
Rhomboids
Rotatores
Semispinalis thoracis
Spinalis thoracis

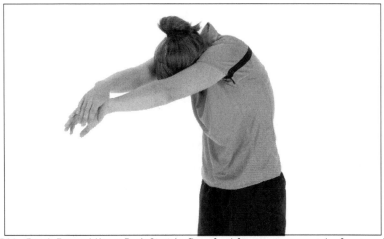

D01 - Reach Forward Upper Back Stretch: Stand with your arms out in front and your hands crossed over, then push your hands forward as far as possible and let your head fall forward.

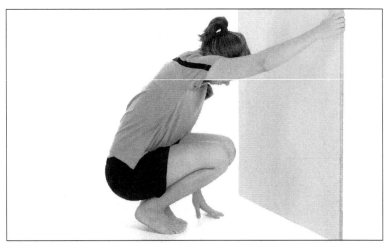

D02 - Reaching Upper Back Stretch: Sit in a squatting position while facing a door edge or pole, then hold onto the door edge with one hand and lean backwards away from the door.

Stretches for the Back and Sides

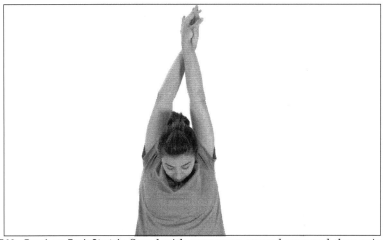

D03 - Reach-up Back Stretch: Stand with your arms crossed over and then raise them above your head. Let your head fall forward and reach up as high as you can.

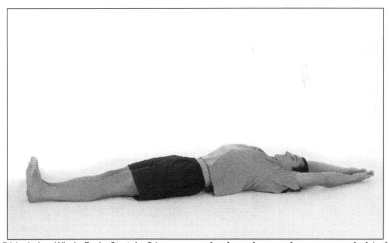

D04 - Lying Whole Body Stretch: Lie on your back and extend your arms behind you. Keep your toes pointing upwards and lengthen your body as much as you can.

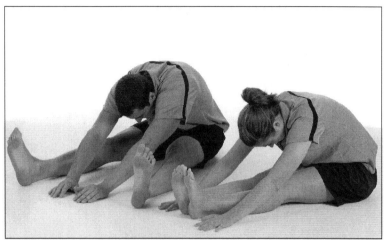

D05 - Sitting Bent-over Back Stretch: Sit on the ground with your legs straight out in front or at 45 degrees apart. Keep your toes pointing upwards and rest your arms by your side or on your lap. Relax your back and neck and let your head and chest fall forward.

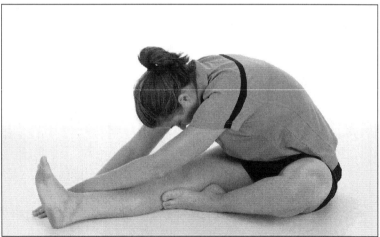

D06 - Sitting Side Reach Stretch: Sit with one leg straight out to the side and your toes pointing upwards. Then bring your other foot up to your knee and let your head fall forward. Reach towards the outside of your toes with both hands.

Stretches for the Back and Sides

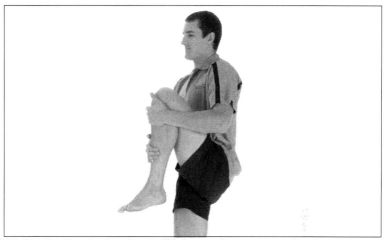

D07 - Standing Knee-to-chest Stretch: While standing, use your hands to bring one knee into your chest.

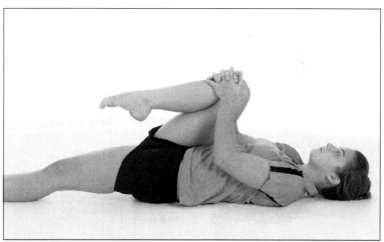

D08 - Lying Knee-to-chest Stretch: Lie on your back and keep one leg flat on the ground. Use your hands to bring your other knee into your chest.

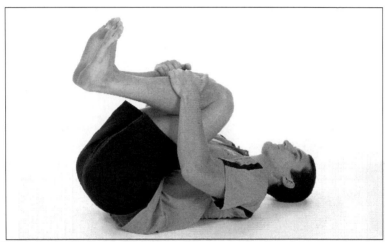

D09 - Lying Double Knee-to-chest Stretch: Lie on your back and use your hands to bring both knees into your chest.

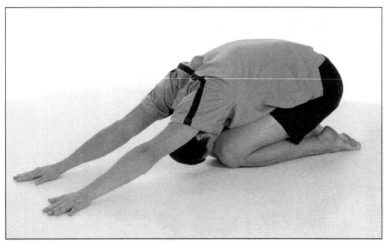

D10 - Kneeling Reach Forward Stretch: Kneel on the ground and reach forward with your hands. Let your head fall forward and push your buttocks back towards your feet.

Stretches for the Back and Sides

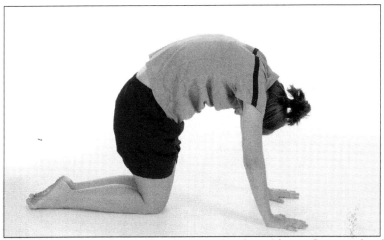

D11 - Kneeling Back-arch Stretch: Kneel on your hands and knees. Let your head fall forward and arch your back upwards.

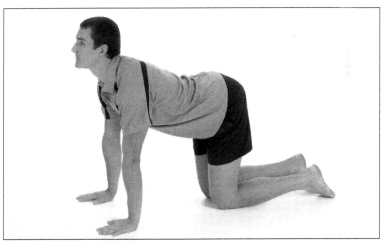

D12 - Kneeling Back-slump Stretch: Kneel on your hands and knees. Look up and let your back slump downwards.

75

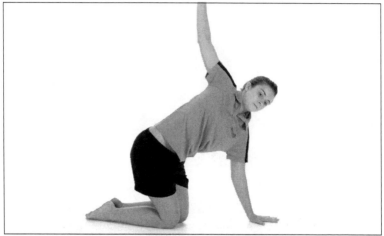

D13 - Kneeling Back Rotation Stretch: Kneel on the ground and raise one arm upwards while rotating your shoulders and middle back.

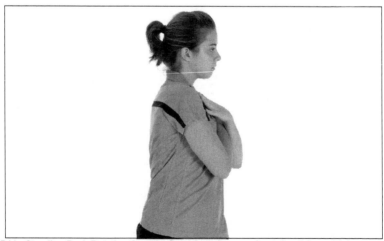

D14 - Standing Back Rotation Stretch: Stand with your feet shoulder width apart. Place your hands across your chest while keeping your back and shoulders upright. Slowly rotate your shoulders to one side.

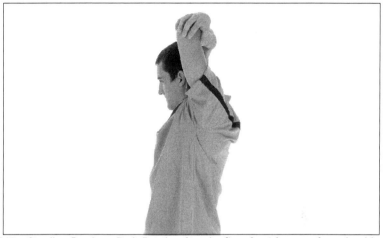

D15 - Standing Reach-up Back Rotation Stretch: Stand with your feet shoulder width apart. Place your hands above your head while keeping your back and shoulders upright. Slowly rotate your back and shoulders to one side.

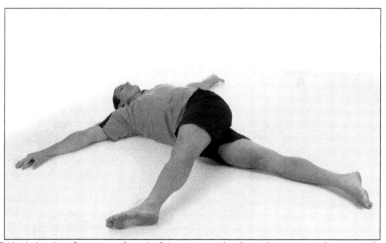

D16 - Lying Leg Cross-over Stretch: Lie on your back and cross one leg over the other. Keep your arms out to the side and both legs straight. Let your back and hips rotate with your leg.

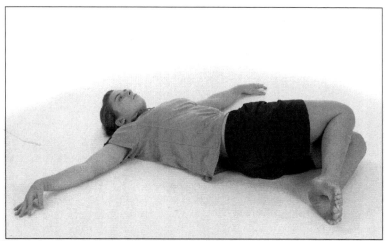

D17 - Lying Knee Roll-over Stretch: While lying on your back, bend your knees and let them fall to one side. Keep your arms out to the side and let your back and hips rotate with your knees.

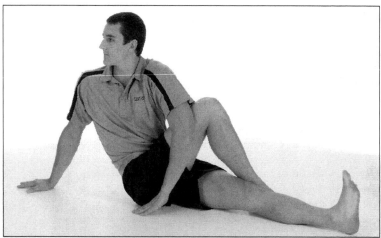

D18 - Sitting Knee-up Rotation Stretch: Sit with one leg straight and the other leg crossed over your knee. Turn your shoulders and put your arm onto your raised knee to help rotate your shoulders and back.

Stretches for the Back and Sides

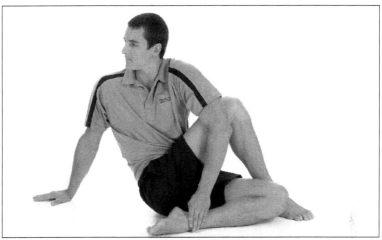

D19 - Sitting knee-up Extended Rotation Stretch: Sit with one leg crossed under the other and the other foot crossed over your knee, then turn your shoulders and put your arm onto your raised knee to help rotate your shoulders and back.

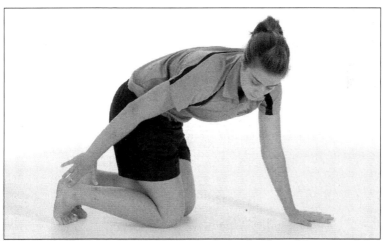

D20 - Kneeling Reach-around Stretch: Kneel on your hands and knees and then take one hand and reach around towards your ankle. Keep your back parallel to the ground.

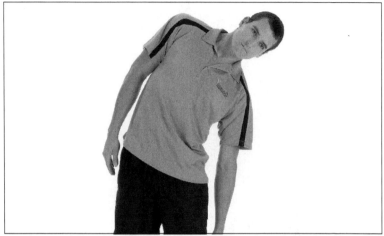

D21 - Standing Lateral Side Stretch: Stand with your feet about shoulder width apart and look forward. Keep your body upright and slowly bend to the left or right. Reach down your leg with your hand and do not bend forward.

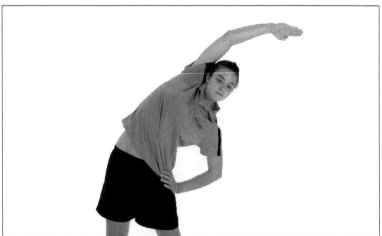

D22 - Reaching Lateral Side Stretch: Stand with your feet shoulder width apart, then slowly bend to the side and reach over the top of your head with your hand. Do not bend forward.

Stretches for the Back and Sides

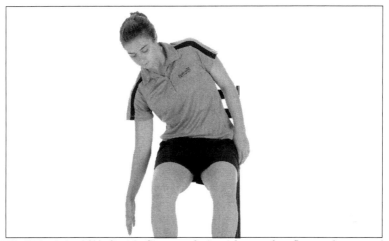

D23 - Sitting Lateral Side Stretch: Sit on a chair with your feet flat on the ground, then slowly bend to the left or right while reaching towards the ground. Do not bend forward.

Stretches for the Hips and Buttocks

The hips and buttocks are comprised of a number of both large muscles (Gluteus maximus) and small muscles (Piriformis). These muscles are primarily responsible for hip stabilization and lower leg movement. The muscles around the hip and buttocks, along with the structure of the hip joint, allow for a large range of motion of the leg; including flexion, extension, adduction, abduction and rotation.

Sports that benefit from these quadriceps stretches include: Cycling; Hiking, Backpacking, Mountaineering and Orienteering; Ice hockey and Field hockey; Ice Skating, Roller Skating and Inline Skating; Martial Arts; Rowing, Canoeing and Kayaking; Running, Track and Cross Country; running sports like Football, Soccer, Gridiron and Rugby; Snow Skiing and Water Skiing; Walking and Race Walking.

The major muscles being stretched.
Gemellus superior and inferior
Gluteus maximus
Iliacus
Obturator internus and externus
Piriformis
Psoas major
Psoas minor
Quadratus femoris

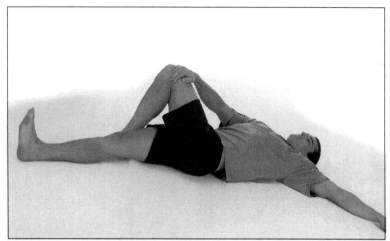

E01 - Lying Cross-over Knee Pull-down Stretch: Lie on your back and cross one leg over the other. Bring your foot up to your opposite knee and with your opposite arm pull your raised knee down towards the ground.

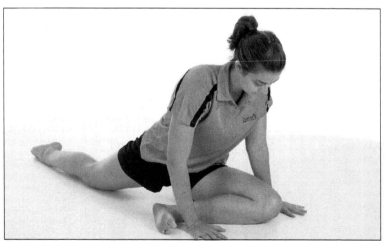

E02 - Lying Leg Tuck Hip Stretch: Lie face down and bend one leg under your stomach. Lean towards the ground.

Stretches for the Hips and Buttocks

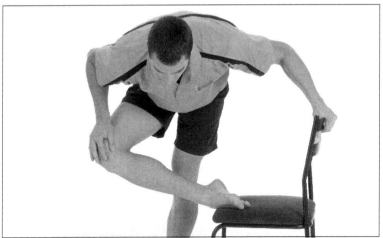

E03 - Standing Leg Tuck Hip Stretch: Stand beside a chair or table and place the foot furthest from the object onto the object. Relax your leg, lean forward and bend your other leg, lowering yourself towards the ground.

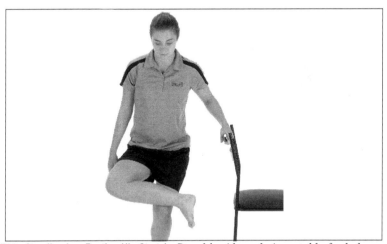

E04 - Standing Leg Resting Hip Stretch: Stand beside a chair or table for balance, bend one leg and place your other ankle on to your bent knee. Slowly lower yourself towards the ground.

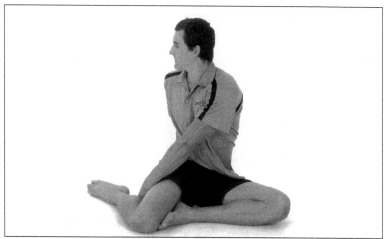

E05 - Sitting Rotational Hip Stretch: Sit with one leg crossed and your other leg behind your buttocks then lean your whole body towards the leg that is behind your buttocks.

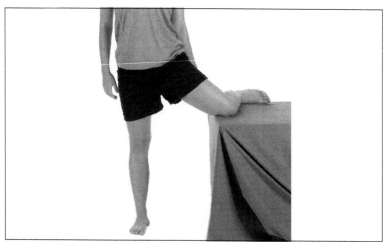

E06 - Standing Rotational Hip Stretch: Stand beside a table and raise your lower leg out to the side and up onto the table. Then slowly lower your body.

Stretches for the Hips and Buttocks

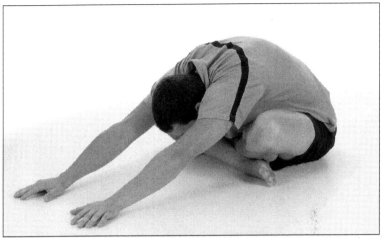

E07 - Sitting Cross-legged Reach Forward Stretch: Sit with your legs crossed and your knees out, and then gently reach forward.

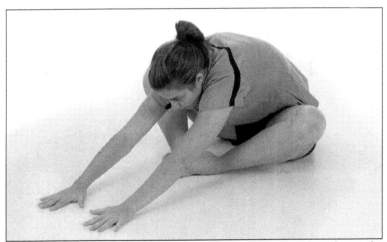

E08 - Sitting Feet-together Reach Forward Stretch: Sit with the soles of your feet together and your knees out, and then gently reach forward.

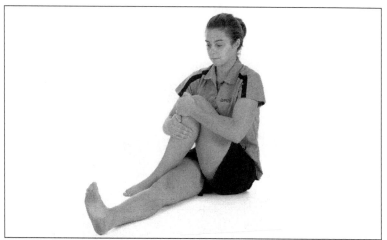

E09 - Sitting Knee-to-chest Buttocks Stretch: Sit with one leg straight and the other leg crossed over your knee. Pull the raised knee towards your opposite shoulder while keeping your back straight and your shoulders facing forward.

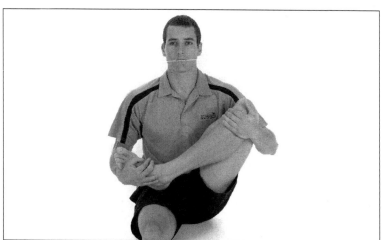

E10 - Sitting Foot-to-chest Buttocks Stretch: Sit with one leg straight, hold onto your other ankle and then pull it directly towards your chest.

Stretches for the Hips and Buttocks

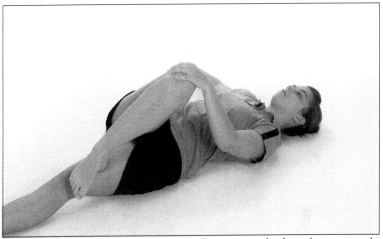

E11 - Lying Cross-over Knee Pull-up Stretch: Lie on your back and cross one leg over the other. Bring your foot up to your opposite knee and with your opposite arm pull your raised knee up towards your chest.

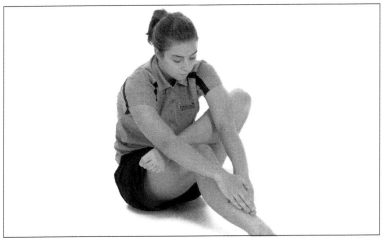

E12 - Sitting Leg Resting Buttocks Stretch: Sit with one leg slightly bent. Raise your other foot up onto your raised leg and rest it on your thigh, then slowly reach forward.

89

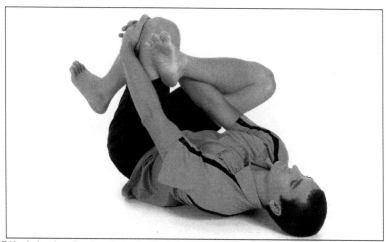

E13 - Lying Leg Resting Buttocks Stretch: Lie on your back and slightly bend one leg. Raise your other foot up onto your bent leg and rest it on your thigh. Then reach forward, holding onto your knee and pull towards you.

Stretches for the Quadriceps

The quadriceps is a large group of muscles located in the anterior (front) of the thigh. They originate from above the hip joint and extend to below the knee. The primary action of the quadriceps is to extend the knee joint, but in conjunction with a number of other muscles in the front of the hip, they are also associated with hip flexion.

The following quadriceps stretches (F02, F04, F05, F06, and F07) place the knee joint into full flexion, which can stress the anatomical structures of the knee joint. If you have a knee injury or suffer from knee pain, take extra care when performing these stretches or avoid them altogether.

Sports that benefit from these quadriceps stretches include: Cycling; Hiking, Backpacking, Mountaineering and Orienteering; Ice Hockey and Field Hockey; Ice Skating, Roller Skating and Inline Skating; Martial Arts; Running, Track and Cross Country; running sports like Football, Soccer, Gridiron and Rugby; Snow Skiing and Water Skiing; Surfing; Walking and Race Walking.

The major muscles being stretched.
Rectus femoris
Sartorius
Vastus intermedius
Vastus lateralis
Vastus medialis

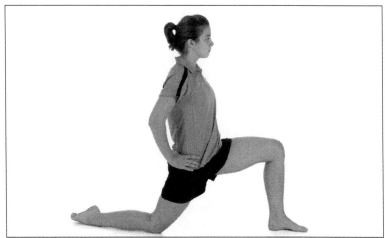

F01 - Kneeling Quad Stretch: Kneel on one foot and the other knee. If needed, hold on to something to keep your balance and then push your hips forward.

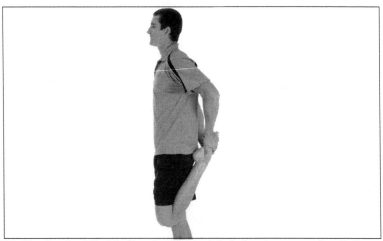

F02 - Standing Quad Stretch: Stand upright while balancing on one leg. Pull your other foot up behind your buttocks and keep your knees together while pushing your hips forward. Hold on to something for balance if needed.

Stretches for the Quadriceps

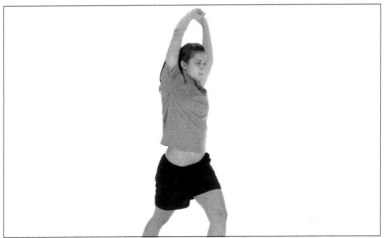

F03 - Standing Reach-up Quad Stretch: Stand upright and take one small step forward. Reach up with both hands, push your hips forward, lean back and then lean away from your back leg.

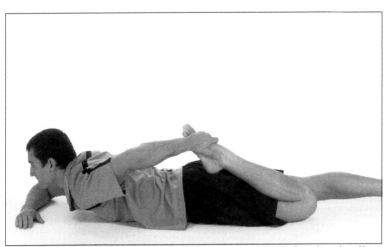

F04 - Lying Quad Stretch: Lie face down, reach back with one hand and pull one foot up behind your buttocks.

93

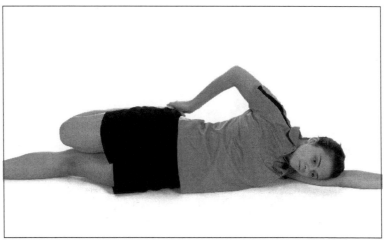

F05 - Lying Side Quad Stretch: Lie on your side and pull your top leg behind your buttocks. Keep your knees together and push your hips forward.

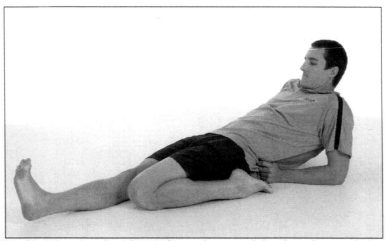

F06 - Single Lean-back Quad Stretch: Sit on the ground, bend one knee and place that foot next to your buttocks. Then slowly lean backwards.

Stretches for the Quadriceps

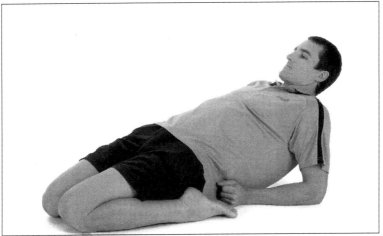

F07 - Double Lean-back Quad Stretch: Sit on the ground, bend both knees and place your feet next to your buttocks. Then slowly lean backwards.

Stretches for the Hamstrings

The hamstrings are a large group of muscles located in the posterior (rear) of the thigh. They originate from the bottom of the hip bone and extend to below the knee. The primary action of the hamstrings is to flex the knee joint.

Sports that benefit from these hamstring stretches include: Basketball and Netball; Cycling; Hiking, Backpacking, Mountaineering and Orienteering; Ice Hockey and Field Hockey; Ice Skating, Roller Skating and Inline Skating; Martial Arts; Running, Track and Cross Country; running sports like Football, Soccer, Gridiron and Rugby; Snow Skiing and Water Skiing; Surfing; Walking and Race Walking; and Wrestling.

The major muscles being stretched.
Biceps femoris
Semimembranosus
Semitendinosis

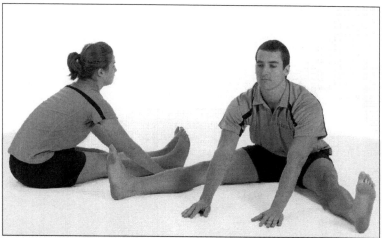

G01 - Sitting Reach-forward Hamstring Stretch: Sit with both legs straight out in front, or at 45 degrees apart. Keep your toes pointing straight up, make sure your back is straight and then reach forward.

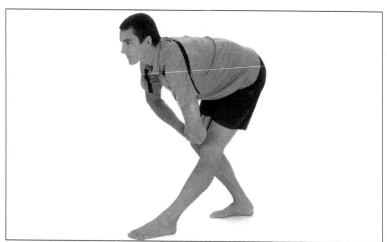

G02 - Standing Toe-down Hamstring Stretch: Stand with one knee bent and the other leg straight out in front. Point your toes towards the ground and lean forward. Keep your back straight and rest your hands on your bent knee.

Stretches for the Hamstrings

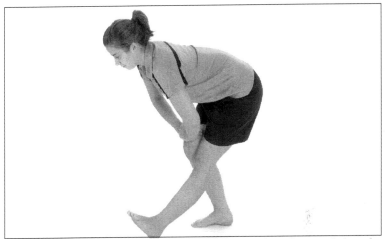

G03 - Standing Toe-up Hamstring Stretch: Stand with one knee bent and the other leg straight out in front. Point your toes upwards and lean forward. Keep your back straight and rest your hands on your bent knee.

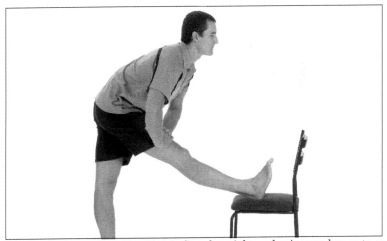

G04 - Standing Leg-up Hamstring Stretch: Stand upright and raise one leg on to an object. Keep that leg straight and point your toes upwards. Keep your back straight and lean your upper body forward.

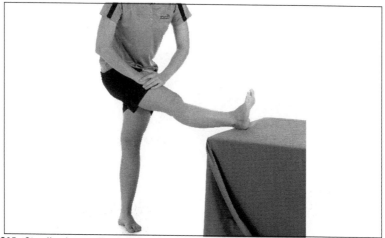

G05 - Standing Leg-up Toe-in Hamstring Stretch: Stand upright and raise one leg on to an object. Keep that leg straight and point your toes upwards. Then point the toes of your other foot inward and lean forward while keeping your back straight.

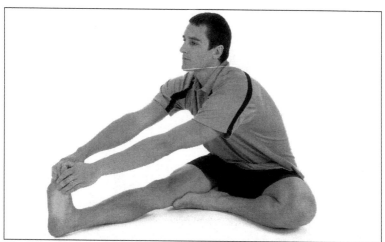

G06 - Sitting Single Leg Hamstring Stretch: Sit with one leg straight out in front and point your toes upwards. Bring your other foot towards your knee and reach towards your toes with both hands.

Stretches for the Hamstrings

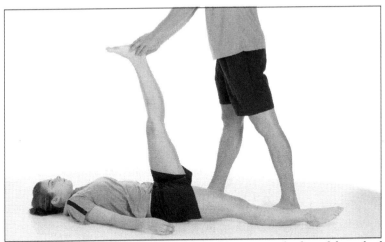

G07 - Lying Partner Assisted Hamstring Stretch: Lie on your back and keep both legs straight. Have a partner raise one of your legs off the ground and as far back as is comfortable. Make sure your toes are pointing directly backwards.

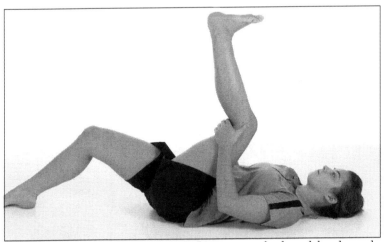

G08 - Lying Bent Knee Hamstring Stretch: Lie on your back and bend one leg slightly. Pull the other knee towards your chest and then slowly straighten your raised leg.

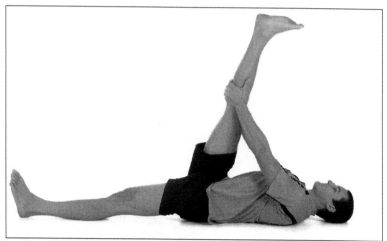

G09 - Lying Straight Knee Hamstring Stretch: Lie on your back and keep your legs straight. Raise one leg and pull it towards your chest.

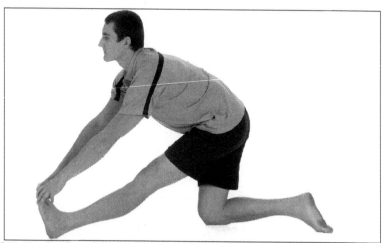

G10 - Kneeling Toe-up Hamstring Stretch: Kneel on one knee and place your other leg straight forward with your heel on the ground. Keep your back straight and point your toes upwards. Reach towards your toes with one or both hand.

Stretches for the Hamstrings

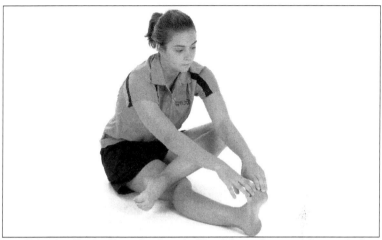

G11 - Sitting Leg Resting Hamstring Stretch: Sit with one leg straight out in front and your toes pointing upwards. Cross your other leg over and rest your foot on your thigh. Lean forward, keep your back straight and reach for your toes.

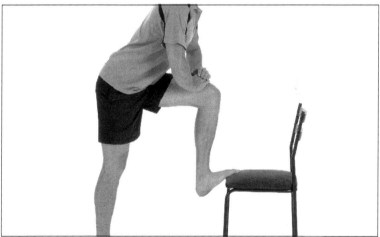

G12 - Standing Leg-up Bent Knee Hamstring Stretch: Stand with one foot raised onto a chair or an object. Bend your knee and let your heel drop off the edge of the object. Keep your back straight and move your chest towards your raised knee.

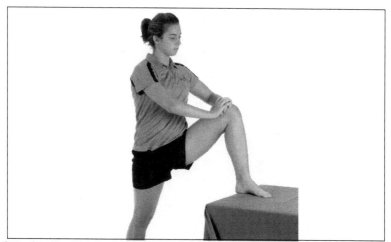

G13 - Standing High-leg Bent Knee Hamstring Stretch: Stand with one foot raised onto a table. Keep your leg bent and lean your chest into your bent knee.

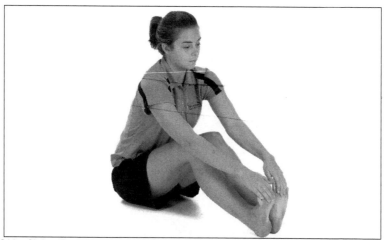

G14 - Sitting Bent Knee Toe-pull Hamstring Stretch: Sit on the ground with your knees slightly bent. Hold onto your toes with your hands and pull your toes towards your body. Keep your back straight and lean forward.

Stretches for the Hamstrings

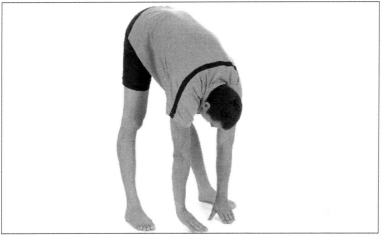

G15 - Standing Reach-down Hamstring Stretch: Stand with your feet shoulder width apart. Bend forward and reach towards the ground.

Stretches for the Adductors

The adductors are a large group of muscles located on the medial (inner) side of the thigh. They originate at the bottom of the hip bone and extend down the inside of the thigh attaching to the medial side of the femur. The primary action of the adductors is to adduct (draw towards the midline) the hip joint.

Sports that benefit from these adductor stretches include: Basketball and Netball; Cycling; Hiking, Backpacking, Mountaineering and Orienteering; Ice Hockey and Field Hockey; Ice Skating, Roller Skating and Inline Skating; Martial Arts; Running, Track and Cross Country; running sports like Football, Soccer, Gridiron and Rugby; Snow Skiing and Water Skiing; Surfing; Walking and Race Walking; and Wrestling.

The major muscles being stretched.

Adductor brevis
Adductor longus
Adductor magnus
Pectineus
Gracilis

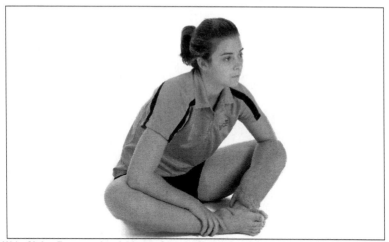

H01 - Sitting Feet-together Adductor Stretch: Sit with the soles of your feet together and bring your feet towards your groin. Hold onto your ankles and push your knees toward the ground with your elbows. Keep your back straight.

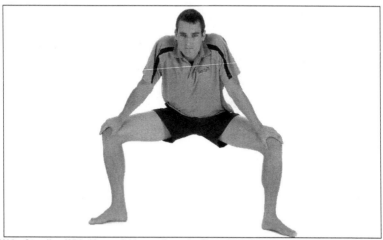

H02 - Standing Wide Knees Adductor Stretch: Stand with your feet wide apart and your toes pointing diagonally outwards, then bend your knees, lean forward and use your hands to push your knees outwards.

Stretches for the Adductors

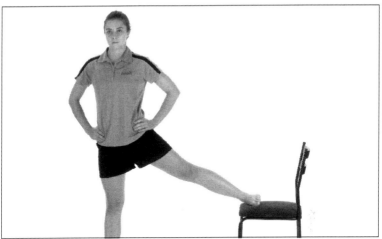

H03 - Standing Leg-up Adductor Stretch: Stand upright and place one leg out to the side and your foot up on a raised object. Keep your toes facing forward and slowly move your other leg away from the object.

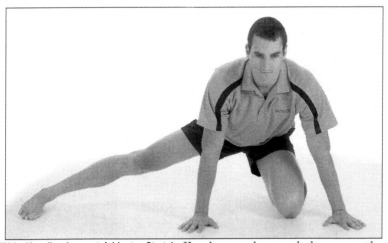

H04 - Kneeling Leg-out Adductor Stretch: Kneel on one knee and place your other leg out to the side with your toes pointing forward. Rest your hands on the ground and slowly move your foot further out to the side.

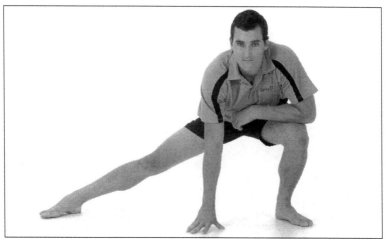

H05 - Squatting Leg-out Adductor Stretch: Stand with your feet wide apart. Keep one leg straight and your toes pointing forward while bending the other leg and turning your toes out to the side. Lower your groin towards the ground and rest your hands on your bent knee or the ground.

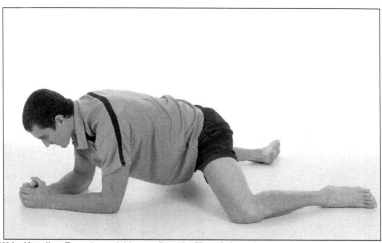

H06 - Kneeling Face-down Adductor Stretch: Kneel face down with your knees and toes facing out. Lean forward and let your knees move outwards.

Stretches for the Adductors

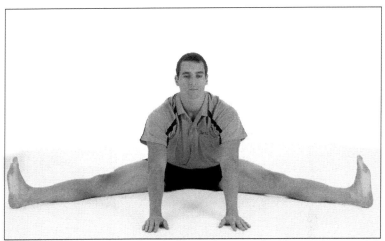

H07 - Sitting Wide-leg Adductor Stretch: Sit on the ground with your legs straight out and as wide apart as possible and then reach forward while keeping your back straight.

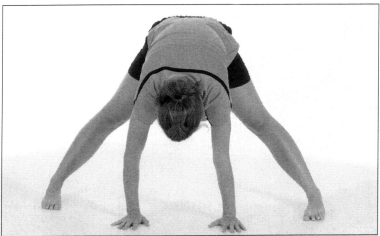

H08 - Standing Wide-leg Adductor Stretch: Start by standing with your feet wide apart and your toes pointing forward. Then lean forward and reach towards the ground.

Stretches for the Abductors

The abductors are located on the lateral side (outside) of the thigh and hip. They originate at the top outer edge of the hip bone and extend down the outside of the thigh attaching to the lateral side of the tibia. The primary action of the abductors is to abduct (draw away from the midline) the hip joint.

Sports that benefit from these abductor stretches include: Cycling; Hiking, Backpacking, Mountaineering and Orienteering; Ice hockey and Field hockey; Ice Skating, Roller Skating and Inline Skating; Martial Arts; Rowing, Canoeing and Kayaking; Running, Track and Cross Country; running sports like Football, Soccer, Gridiron and Rugby; Snow Skiing and Water Skiing; Walking and Race Walking.

The major muscles being stretched.
Gluteus medius
Gluteus mininus
Tensor fasciae latae

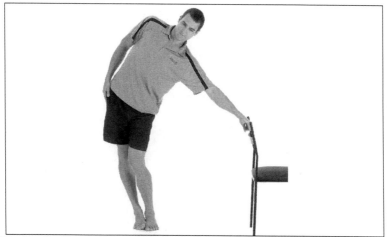

I01 - Standing Hip-out Abductor Stretch: Stand upright beside a chair or table with both feet together. Lean your upper body towards the chair while pushing your hips away from the chair. Keep your outside leg straight and bend your inside leg slightly.

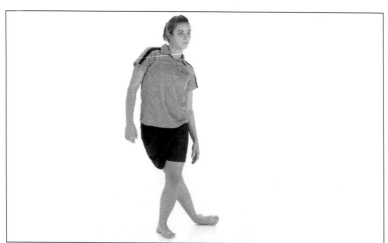

I02 - Standing Leg-cross Abductor Stretch: Stand upright and cross one foot behind the other. Lean towards the foot that is behind the other.

Stretches for the Abductors

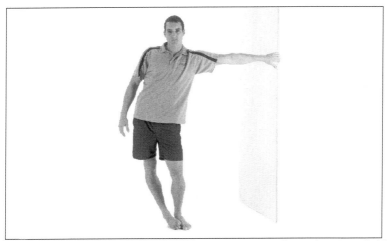

103 - Leaning Abductor Stretch: While standing next to a pole, or door jam, hold onto the pole with one hand. Keep your feet together, and lean your hips away from the pole. Keep your outside leg straight and bend your inside leg slightly.

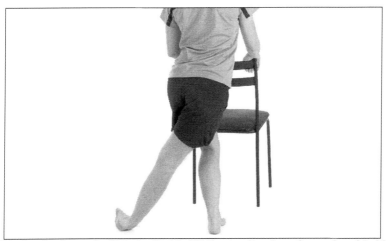

104 - Standing Leg-under Abductor Stretch: While standing lean forward and hold onto a chair or bench to help with balance. Cross one foot behind the other and slide that foot to the side. Keep your leg straight and slowly bend your front leg to lower your body.

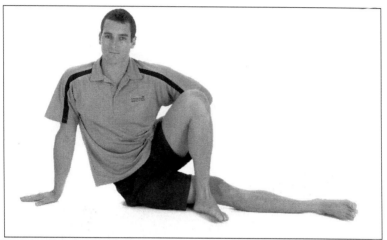

105 - Lying Abductor Stretch: Lean on your side on the ground and bring your top leg up to your other knee. Push your body up with your arm and keep your hip on the ground.

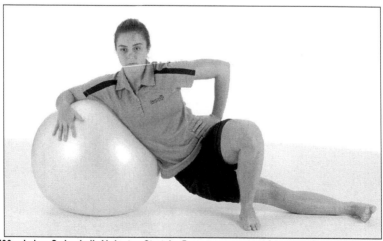

106 - Lying Swiss-ball Abductor Stretch: Lean on your side on a Swiss ball and place one leg straight out to the side. Bring your top leg up to your other knee and push your hip towards the ground.

Stretches for the Abductors

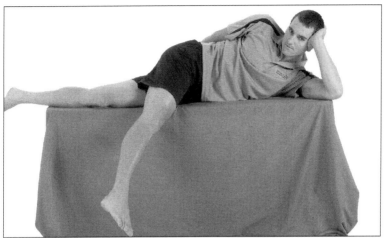

107 - Lying Leg-hang Abductor Stretch: Lie on your side on a bench, let your top leg fall forward and off the side of the bench.

Stretches for the Upper Calves

The upper calf muscles are located on the posterior (rear) of the lower leg just underneath the knee joint. They originate at the bottom of the femur, just above the knee joint, and extend down into the Achilles tendon. The primary actions of the upper calf muscles are to plantar flex the ankle joint and flex the knee.

The calf muscles and Achilles tendon are commonly over-stretched by applying too much force to the targeted muscle groups. Please take extra care when performing the following stretches and always follow *The Rules for Safe Stretching* in chapter 5.

Sports that benefit from these upper calf stretches include: Basketball and Netball; Boxing; Cycling; Hiking, Backpacking, Mountaineering and Orienteering; Ice hockey and Field hockey; Ice Skating, Roller Skating and Inline Skating; Martial Arts; racquet sports like Tennis, Badminton and Squash; Running, Track and Cross Country; running sports like Football, Soccer, Gridiron and Rugby; Snow Skiing and Water Skiing; Surfing; Swimming; Walking and Race Walking.

The major muscles being stretched.
Gastrocnemius
Plantaris

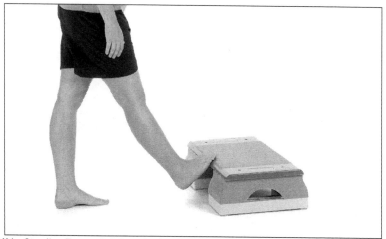

J01 - Standing Toe-up Calf Stretch: Stand upright and place the ball of your foot on a step or raised object. Keep your leg straight and lean towards your toes.

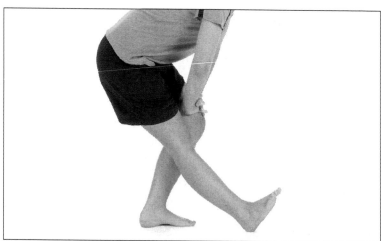

J02 - Standing Toe Raised Calf Stretch: Stand with one knee bent and the other leg straight out in front. Point your toes upwards and lean forward. Keep your back straight and rest your hands on your bent knee.

Stretches for the Upper Calves

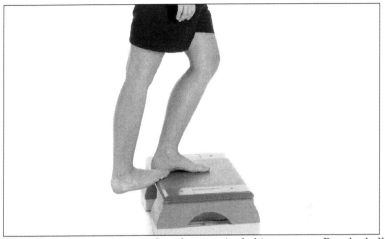

J03 - Single Heel-drop Calf Stretch: Stand on a raised object or step. Put the ball of one foot on the edge of the step and keep your leg straight. Let your heel drop towards the ground.

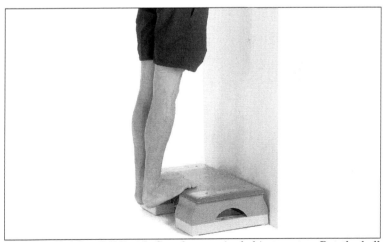

J04 - Double Heel-drop Calf Stretch: Stand on a raised object or step. Put the balls of both feet on the edge of the step and keep your legs straight. Let your heels drop towards the ground.

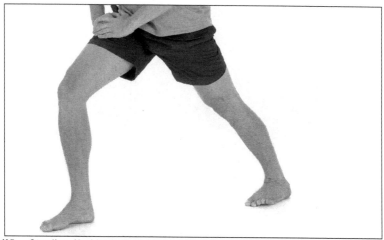

J05 - Standing Heel-back Calf Stretch: Stand upright and take one big step backwards. Keep your back leg straight, your toes pointing forward and push your heel to the ground.

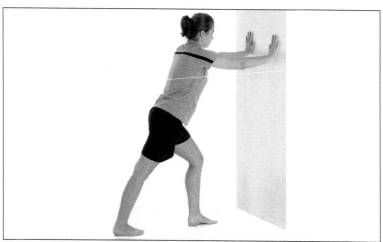

J06 - Leaning Heel-back Calf Stretch: Reach towards a wall and place one foot as far from the wall as is comfortable. Make sure that both toes are pointing forward and your heel is on the ground. Keep your back leg straight and lean towards the wall.

Stretches for the Upper Calves

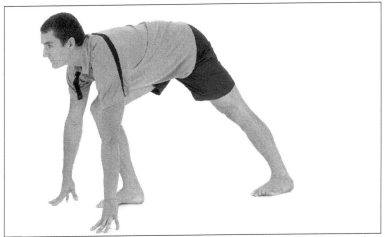

J07 - Crouching Heel-back Calf Stretch: Stand upright and place one foot in front of the other. Bend your front leg and keep your back leg straight. Push your heel to the ground and lean forward. Place your hands on the ground in front of you.

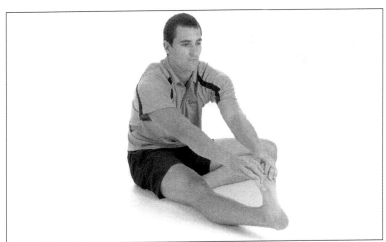

J08 - Sitting Toe-pull Calf Stretch: Sit with one leg straight out in front and your toes pointing upwards. Reach forward and pull your toes back towards your body.

Stretches for the Lower Calves and Achilles

The lower calf muscles are located on the posterior (rear) of the lower leg below the knee joint. They originate at the top of the tibia, just below the knee joint, and extend down into the Achilles tendon. The primary action of the lower calf muscles is to plantar flex the ankle joint.

The calf muscles and Achilles tendon are commonly over-stretched by applying too much force to the targeted muscle groups. Please take extra care when performing the following stretches and always follow *The Rules for Safe Stretching* in chapter 5.

Sports that benefit from these lower calf stretches include: Basketball and Netball; Boxing; Cycling; Hiking, Backpacking, Mountaineering and Orienteering; Ice hockey and Field hockey; Ice Skating, Roller Skating and Inline Skating; Martial Arts; racquet sports like Tennis, Badminton and Squash; Running, Track and Cross Country; running sports like Football, Soccer, Gridiron and Rugby; Snow Skiing and Water Skiing; Surfing; Swimming; Walking and Race Walking.

The major muscles being stretched.
Flexor digitorum longus
Flexor hallucis longus
Peroneus longus and brevis
Soleus
Tibialis posterior

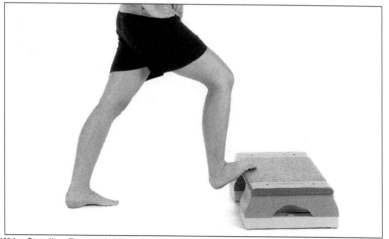

K01 - Standing Toe-up Achilles Stretch: Stand upright and place the ball of your foot onto a step or raised object. Bend your knee and lean forward.

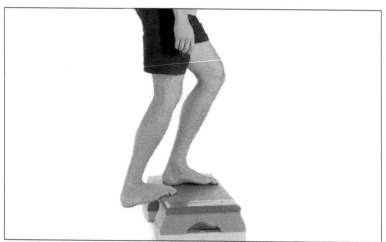

K02 - Single Heel-drop Achilles Stretch: Stand on a raised object or step and place the ball of one of your feet on the edge of the step. Bend your knee slightly and let your heel drop towards the ground.

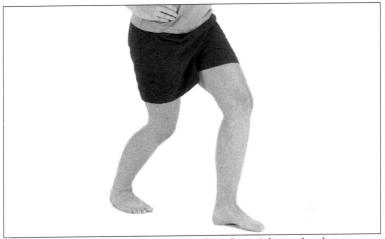

K03 - Standing Heel-back Achilles Stretch: Stand upright and take one step backwards. Bend your back knee and push your heel towards the ground.

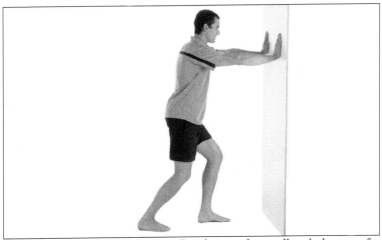

K04 - Leaning Heel-back Achilles Stretch: Reach towards a wall and place one foot as far from the wall as is comfortable. Make sure that both toes are pointing forward and your heels are on the ground. Bend your back knee and lean towards the wall.

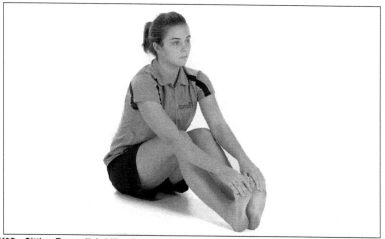

K05 - Sitting Toe-pull Achilles Stretch: Sit on the ground with your knees slightly bent. Hold onto your toes with your hands and pull your toes towards your body.

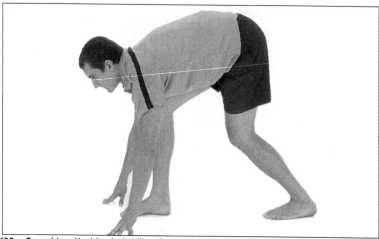

K06 - Crouching Heel-back Achilles Stretch: Stand upright and place one foot in front of the other. Bend your front leg and your back leg and then push your back heel towards the ground. Lean forward and place your hands on the ground in front of you.

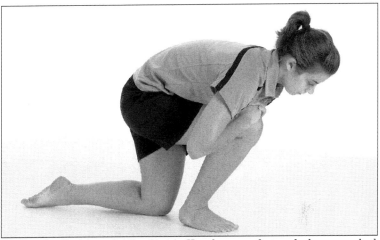

K07 - Kneeling Heel-down Achilles Stretch: Kneel on one foot and place your body weight over your knee. Keep your heel on the ground and lean forward.

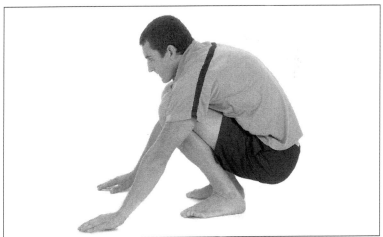

K08 - Squatting Achilles Stretch: Stand with your feet shoulder width apart. Then bend your legs and lower your body into a sitting position. Place your hands out in front for balance.

Stretches for the Shins, Ankles, Feet and Toes

The muscles of the shin originate at the top of the tibia, just below the knee joint, and extend down the front of the shin and over the ankle joint. The primary action of the shin muscles is to dorsiflex the ankle joint.

The feet and ankles are comprised of a multitude of small muscles that control the foot. The muscles around the feet and ankles, along with the structure of the joints, allow for a large range of motion of the feet and ankle; including plantar flexion, dorsiflexion, inversion, eversion and rotation.

Sports that benefit from these shin, ankles and feet stretches include: Basketball and Netball; Boxing; Cycling; Hiking, Backpacking, Mountaineering and Orienteering; Ice hockey and Field hockey; Ice Skating, Roller Skating and Inline Skating; Martial Arts; racquet sports like Tennis, Badminton and Squash; Running, Track and Cross Country; running sports like Football, Soccer, Gridiron and Rugby; Snow Skiing and Water Skiing; Surfing; Swimming; Walking and Race Walking.

The major muscles being stretched.
Abductor digiti minimi
Abductor hallucis
Adductor hallucis
Extensor digitorum longus
Extensor hallucis longus
Flexor digiti minimi brevis
Quadratus plantae
Tibialis anterior

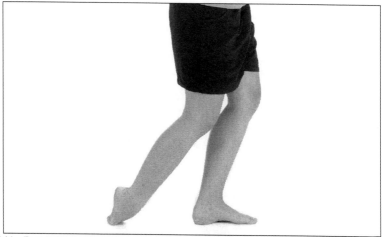

L01 - Foot-behind Shin Stretch: Stand upright and place the top of your toes on the ground behind you. Push your ankle to the ground.

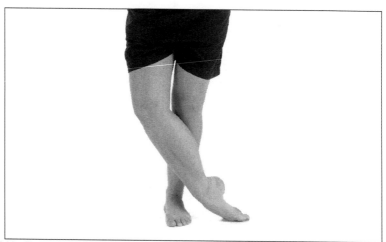

L02 - Front Cross-over Shin Stretch: Stand upright and place the top of your toes on the ground in front of your other foot. Slowly bend your other knee to force your ankle to the ground.

Stretches for the Shins, Ankles, Feet and Toes

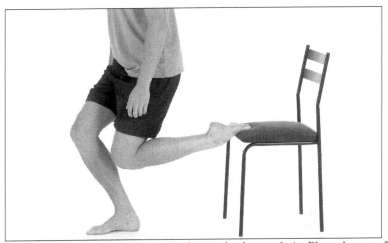

L03 - Raised Foot Shin Stretch: Stand with your back to a chair. Place the top of your toes onto the chair and then push your ankle downwards.

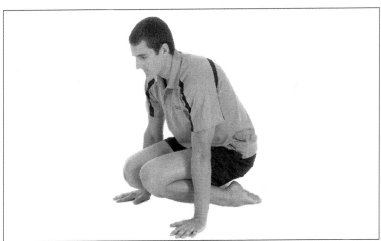

L04 - Double Kneeling Shin Stretch: Sit with your knees and feet flat on the ground. Sit back on your ankles and keep your knees together. Place your hands next to your knees and slowly lean backwards while raising your knees off the ground.

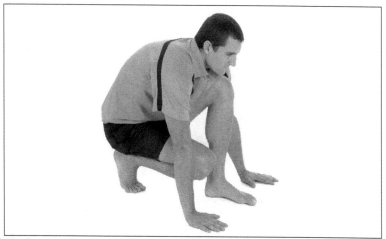

L05 - Squatting Toe Stretch: Kneel on one foot with your hands on the ground. Keep the toes of your rear foot on the ground, slowly lean forward and arch your foot.

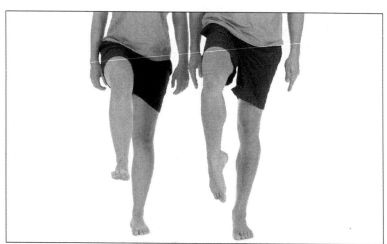

L06 - Ankle Rotation Stretch: Raise one foot off the ground and slowly rotate your foot and ankle in all directions.

Top 5 Stretches for each Sport

The stretches below are a short list of some of the most beneficial stretches for each sport. Obviously there are a lot more, but these are a great place to start.

Sports	Stretches
Archery	A16, B12, C02, D06, D14
Basketball	A05, B13, F03, H05, K07
Backpacking	C02, D11, E07, G03, K07
Batting sports:	
(Cricket, Baseball, Softball, etc.)	A09, B16, C03, D02, D18
Boxing	A01, A07, B08, B17, D17
Canoeing	A13, A16, B06, D20, E04
Contact sports:	
(Football, Gridiron, Rugby, etc.)	A02, A07, E08, F01, H05
Cross Country	C05, F03, I04, K07, L01
Cycling	B06, D08, E05, F05, J03
Field Hockey	D22, E07, F02, H04, J02
Golf	A17, B12, D06, D18, I04
Gridiron	D13, E10, F06, G13, H02
Hiking	C03, D11, E03, G01, J03
Ice Hockey	D23, E08, F01, H02, K07
Ice Skating	D07, E03, E12, F01, H01
Inline Skating	D09, E04, E10, F03, H04
Kayaking	A13, A17, B07, D18, E03
Martial Arts	B17, C05, D13, G05, H06
Mountaineering	C02, D09, E01, G03, L02
Netball	A02, B14, F03, H05, K04
Orienteering	C03, D13, E04, G06, K02
Race walking	D17, E05, F03, J02, K04
Racquet sports:	
(Tennis, Badminton, Squash, etc.)	A14, B07, B17, C03, D16
Roller Skating	D08, E04, E13, F06, H03
Rowing	A15, A16, B06, C05, E01
Running	C03, F01, G04, I02, K04
Rugby	D17, E04, F01, G04, H05
Snow Boarding	D13, E01, E13, F01, I04
Snow Skiing	D06, D22, F06, I03, K07
Soccer	F01, G05, H05, J06, L02
Surfing	C05, D16, E07, F05, I02

Swimming	A12, A14, B08, D04, J03
Throwing sports:	
(Cricket, Baseball, Field Events, etc.)	A13, A17, B14, B17, D18
Volleyball	A12, D22, E10, H02, K07
Walking	D21, E08, F05, J03, K01
Water skiing	B01, C03, D10, E09, F06
Wrestling	D15, D22, E06, G01, H06

Top 5 Stretches for each Sports Injury

The stretches below are a short list of suggested stretches to help with a number of common sports injuries. The following stretches are beneficial for the prevention and long term rehabilitation of the injuries listed below; however, they are not to be used in the initial stages of injury rehabilitation. Stretching during this early stage of the rehabilitation process can cause more damage to the injured tissues. **Avoid all stretching during the first 72 hours after any soft tissue injury**, and remember to follow *The Rules for Safe Stretching* in chapter 5.

Sports Injury	Stretches
Head and Neck	
Whiplash & Wryneck	A01, A02, A04, A07, A11
Hands and Fingers	
Thumb Sprain	B12, B13, B14, B15, B17
Finger Sprain & Tendinitis	B11, B12, B13, B14, B17
Wrists and Forearm	
Wrist Sprain & Tendinitis	B04, B11, B12, B16, B17
Carpel Tunnel & Ulnar Tunnel Syndrome	B02, B11, B13, B16, B17
Elbow	
Elbow Sprain	A08, A16, B10, B11, B17
Triceps Tendon Rupture	A09, B01, B06, B09, B10
Tennis, Golfers & Throwers Elbow	A12, A14, A16, B01, B10
Shoulder and Upper Arm	
Biceps Bruise, Strain & Tendinitis	A17, B02, B06, B07, B11
Chest Strain	A14, A17, B04, B05, B07
Pectoral Muscle Insertion Inflammation	A14, B01, B04, B05, B07
Impingement Syndrome	A16, B01, B06, B07, B10
Rotator Cuff Tendinitis	A09, A12, A13, A14, A15
Frozen Shoulder *(Adhesive Capsulitis)*	A08, A14, A16, B06, B07
Back and Spine	
Muscle Bruise & Strain	D05, D08, D13, D18, D22
Ligament Sprain	D01, D05, D09, D14, D21

Abdomen
Muscle Strain   C02, C03, C05, D14, D21

Hips, Pelvis and Groin
Hip Flexor Strain & Iliopsoas Tendinitis   C03, F01, F02, F03, F05
Groin Strain & Tendinitis   H01, H02, H04, H06, H08
Osteitis Pubis   G04, G13, H02, H05, H07
Piriformis Syndrome   E01, E03, E05, E09, E11

Hamstrings and Quadriceps
Quadriceps Bruise, Strain & Tendinitis   C05, F01, F02, f05, F06
Hamstring Strain   G01, G05, G08, G11, J03
Iliotibial B& Syndrome   D22, I02, I03, I05, I07

Knee
Medial Collateral Ligament Sprain *(MCL)*   F03, F05, H02, H04, H07
Anterior Cruciate ligament Sprain *(ACL)*   F01, F02, F03, G03, J03
Osgood-Schlatter Syndrome   C03, F02, F03, F04, F06
Patellofemerol Pain Syndrome   F01, F02, F05, H05, I04
Patellar Tendinitis *(Jumpers Knee)*   F02, F03, F06, H04, I02

Lower Leg
Calf Strain   G03, G13, J03, J06, K02
Achilles Tendon Strain & Tendinitis   K01, K02, K04, K05, K07
Shin Splints *(MTSS)*   J06, K02, K04, K07, L02
Anterior Compartment Syndrome   F02, L02, L03, L04, L06

Ankle and Feet
Ankle Sprain   J03, J06, K04, L02, L06
Posterior Tibial Tendinitis   H08, J02, K01, K04, K07
Peroneal Tendinitis   J04, K02, K04, L02, L06
Plantar Fasciitis   J03, J06, K04, K07, L05

Resources

Adler, S. Beckers, D. Buck, M.: 2003. *PNF in Practice*. Springer. NY, USA.

Alter, M.J.: 2004. *Science of Flexibility*. Human Kinetics. IL, USA.

Anderson, R. A.: 2010. *Stretching*. Shelter Publications. CA, USA.

Appleton, B.D.: 1998. *Stretching and Flexibility*. Self Published.

Armiger, P.: 2010. *Stretching for Functional Flexibility*. Lippincott Williams & Wilkins. MD, USA.

Bahr, R. & Maehlum, S.: 2004. *Clinical Guide to Sports Injuries*. Human Kinetics. IL, USA.

Beachle, T. & Earle, R.: 2008. *Essentials of Strength Training and Conditioning*. Human Kinetics. IL, USA.

Chek, P.: 2009. *An Integrated Approach to Stretching*. C.H.E.K. Institute. CA, USA.

Delavier, F.: 2010. *Strength Training Anatomy*. Human Kinetics. IL, USA.

Gummerson. T.: 1990. *Mobility Training for the Martial Arts*. A & C Black. London, UK.

Jarmey, C.: 2003. *The Concise Book of Muscles*. Lotus Publishing. Chichester, UK. www.MuscleAnatomyPictures.com

Jarmey, C.: 2006. *The Concise Book of the Moving Body*. Lotus Publishing. Chichester, UK.

Kurz, T.: 2003. *Stretching Scientifically*. Stadion Publishing Company. VT, USA.

Martini, F. & Timmons, M. & Tallitsch, R.: 2009. *Human Anatomy*. Pearson Benjamin Cummings CA, USA.

Mattes, A.: 2000. *Active Isolated Stretching: The Mattes Method*. Self Published. FL, USA.

McAtee, R. & Charland, J.: 2007. *Facilitated Stretching*. Human Kinetics. IL, USA.

Taylor, KL. Sheppard, JM. Lee, H. Plummer, N.: Negative effect of static stretching restored when combined with a sports specific warm-up component. *Journal of Science and Medicine in Sport*, 2009 Nov; 12(6):657-61.

Tortora, G.J. & Derrickson, B.: 2009. *Principles of Anatomy and Physiology*. John Wiley & Sons, Inc. NJ, USA.

Walker, B.: 2011. *Anatomy of Stretching*. Lotus Publishing. Chichester, UK. www.AnatomyOfStretching.com

Walker, B.: 2007. *Anatomy of Sports Injuries*. Lotus Publishing. Chichester, UK.

Weldon, S.M.: The efficacy of stretching for prevention of exercise-related injury: a systematic review of the literature. *Manual Therapy*, 2003 Volume 8, Issue 3, Page 141.

Wharton, J & P.: 1996. *The Whartons' Stretch Book*. Three Rivers Press. NY, USA.

Ylinen, J.: 2008. *Stretching Therapy*. Elsevier. PA, USA.

About the Author

Brad Walker
Brad is an internationally recognized stretching and sports injury consultant with over 20 years of practical experience in the health and fitness industry. Brad is a Health Science graduate of the University of New England with postgraduate accreditations in athletics, swimming and triathlon coaching. Brad has worked with elite level and world champion athletes and lectures for Sports Medicine Australia on injury prevention.

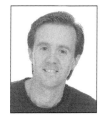

About the Models

Dustin Smith
Dustin is a Level I Artistic Gymnastics coach with over 6 years of professional coaching experience. He holds a Certificate II and III in sport and recreation and is Head Coach & Coordinator of men's gymnastics at the Gold Coast Gymnastics Club in Queensland, Australia. His sporting achievements include state representation for soccer and baseball, and a 3rd place finish for trampoline at the Queensland championships.

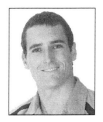

Shannon Austin
Shannon has 14 years of gymnastics competition experience with numerous national and international rankings; including a Level 10 National and State ranking; and a 1st place Level 9 ranking at the 2006 International Hawaii Aloha Gymfest. She currently works as a gymnastics coach at the Gold Coast Gymnastics Club in Queensland, Australia and is studying Secondary Education and PE at university.

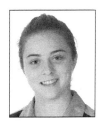

Need help designing a stretching routine?

Designing the right stretching routine isn't easy. Even with a publication like the Ultimate Guide to Stretching & Flexibility, you still need to have a detailed understanding of anatomy and physiology; have experience in basic strength and conditioning techniques; and know precisely which stretches are relevant for each particular muscle group and each particular sport.

And even if you do have all the above, it takes time, discipline and a lot of effort to design and create a safe, effective stretching routine for yourself or your clients.

So, how would you like to have Brad Walker, author of the Ultimate Guide to Stretching & Flexibility, available 24-7 to design stretching routines just for you? Well, now you can! With *InstantStretch* you can access Brad's vast experience and expertise to...

Create as many Professional Stretching Routines as you want, Quickly and Easily - Guaranteed!

With a simple four-step process, *InstantStretch* produces a list of stretches with foolproof, step-by-step instructions and pictures. You can then select, save, print, or email any of the suggested stretching routines.

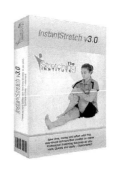

InstantStretch comes complete with over 130 different stretching exercises and creates advanced stretching routines for warming up, cooling down, preventing injury or improving performance. With *InstantStretch* you can create professional stretching routines for over 35 sports and 20 different muscle groups.

For more information, visit...

InstantStretch.com

Your Special Un-Advertised Bonus and Thank-You Gift is FREE!

A short time ago I caught up with a good friend of mine; Christopher Guerriero. He's the author of *Maximize Your Metabolism* and the founder of the National Metabolic & Longevity Research Center in the US, and helps actors, actresses, models and "C" level executives reach their full potential both physically and mentally.

Anyway, we got to talking and he said a lot of his clients had been asking about stretching, and could I do an exclusive audio recording for his clients?

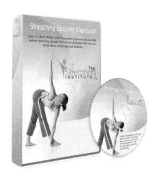

Well, of course I agreed but with one condition; I had to be able to offer the recording to my valued customers. He agreed; and now you can get our exclusive, one-on-one audio recording for free; the same recording that his clients have to pay $97 a month to access.

In this 1 hour MP3 audio presentation, Christopher and I go way beyond the basics and discuss little known stretching secrets that will revolutionize the way you think about stretching and flexibility.

And as a way of saying thank you for purchasing the Ultimate Guide to Stretching & Flexibility, it's yours absolutely free!

Simply visit the web site below and you can listen to the recording online, download the MP3 to your iPod or read the entire word-for-word transcript. I hope you enjoy it.

StretchingSecretsExposed.com